I0022192

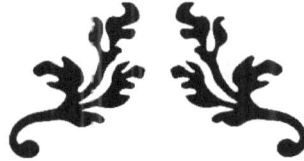

PAIN FREE FUNCTIONAL STRENGTH

Finally, a workout that delivers great results with almost no pain or risk of injury

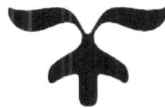

By Michael Spotts: MA. Exercise Physiology

Copyright

Copyright © 2023 by Michael Spotts

All rights reserved. No part of this publication may be reproduced, distributed, or transmitted in any form or by any means, including photocopying, recording, or other electronic or mechanical methods, without the prior written permission of the publisher, except in the case of brief quotations embodied in critical reviews and certain other noncommercial uses permitted by copyright law. For permission requests, write to the publisher, addressed "Attention: Permissions Coordinator," at the address below

Mike Spotts,
1331 Saxon Drive,
Suite 133,
New Smyrna Beach,
Florida, 32169

Painfreefunctionalstrength.com

Ordering Information:
Quantity sales. Special discounts are available on quantity purchases by corporations, associations, and others. For details, contact the publisher at the address above.

Printed in the United States of America

ISBN-13 : 979-8218364366
Pain Free Functional Strength

Disclaimer:

All material in this publication is provided for your information only and may not be construed as medical advice or instruction. No action or inaction should be taken based solely on the contents of this information; instead, readers should consult appropriate health professionals on any matter relating to their health and well-being.

The information and opinions expressed here are believed to be accurate, based on the best judgment available to the author, and readers who fail to consult with appropriate health authorities assume the risk of any injuries. The author acknowledges occasional differences in opinion and welcomes the exchange of different viewpoints.

Preface

Pain Free Functional Strength is a workout for the rest of us, as will be explained later in this book. It was developed after many years of trying and perfecting different ideas with one thing in mind, getting you the user the very best results possible with almost no risk of injury. As you read through this manual, be thinking of how you will use this knowledge to take yourself to new heights in looking and feeling your very best. Once you learn the *Pain Free Functional Strength* methodology, you will have a workout that will serve you well for the rest of your life. No longer will you have to wonder if you're doing the right thing in the gym. Now you will have a program to follow that will get you great results; the same program that has worked for dozens of some of the world's most elite athletes in their fields.

In this manual you will get a thorough explanation of the *Pain Free Functional Strength* You will learn how this program produces great results. It explains in detail all the nuances you will need to know before starting that first workout. You will then find 6 different workouts for all levels of experience in the gym, from the very beginner, to those who have spent many years, or even decades, working out. If you're just starting out you can progress from the beginner workout to the intermediate, and finally to the advanced workout. As you gain confidence with the program, and see the great results you can get, you will find that you can make up your own *Pain Free Functional Strength* workout programs. You will also find blank *Pain Free Functional Strength* workout charts at the end of this manual. Feel free to copy these for your own use after having made your purchase of this publication.

Throughout this book you will read the accounts of real people. Their names and some of the details have been changed for privacy reasons. The results documented are real recordings of their transformative experiences with my program.

Also, the name *Pain Free Functional Strength* was developed within the past few years, and the workout itself has been the result of many years of tweaking and perfecting. For that reason, if you were to ask one of these people about their *Pain Free Functional Strength* workout, they would not be familiar with that name.

I strongly urge you to give this workout your best effort; you will be so very glad you did.

Table of Contents

Glossary of terms

Bar: Curl

The curl bar is a common piece of equipment found in almost all gyms.
It has a distinct bend in it which allows for a more anatomically friendly grip for doing exercises like bicep curls. They typically weigh from 16 to 20 pounds depending on the brand.

Bar: Straight

The larger sized straight bar is also one of most common items found in gyms and is often seen being used for squats and the bench press. These weigh 45 pounds, but if you want to know the exact weight you can lift, be careful. The weight is supposed to be exact, but they almost never are, varying as much as 5 pounds. If you want to know exactly what the weight is, such as for competition, then you must use certified exact weights such as the brand Ivanko. There are also smaller straight bars that weigh about 35 pounds, but these are less common.

Cardiovascular Exercise

This is another type of exercise separate from the ***Pain Free Functional Strength*** program. Briefly, this form of exercise means working in some form of steady, rhythmical method that raises your heart rate and breathing above resting and keeps it there for several minutes. Common forms of this type of exercise are walking, jogging, rowing, in line skating, swimming, and aerobic dance.

Dumbbells

These are individual handheld weights that range normally from 5 pounds to 100 pounds in 5-pound increments.

Free Weights

This term is the most commonly used word for the weights in gyms that include the bars, plates and dumbbells.

Heavy weights junkie

These are people who seem to have to lift the heaviest weights possible almost every time they go to the gym. If this methodology brought great results that would be one thing, but often these folks have chronic injuries and pains that nag them for most of their lives. Somewhere along the line they lost the common sense perspective that working out was actually supposed to make you feel better, not put you in a state of perpetual injury and pain.

Plates

This refers to the circular plate shaped pieces of steel that come in various sizes. The most common sizes are 2 ½, 5, 10, 25, 35, 45, and sometimes even 100 pounds and they are placed on the bars evenly on both sides.

Pain Free Functional Strength

The name of an exercise program carefully and scientifically created for maximum results in looking and feeling your best with the least chance of injury.

Pain Free Functional Strength Cycle

This means that you have gone through the entire program from start to finish. You started by finding just the right weights to start out with and then went for several weeks or months until you could no longer do the number or reps that the program called for on all the exercises.

Pain Free Functional Strength Round

(Used the same as the word "cycle" with the exact same meaning.)

Reps

This is the shortened word for "repetitions". It refers to doing a weightlifting exercise one time. The word rep is almost always used as a group of lifts done in a row. For example, if you are doing an exercise like squats, you can do one set of 10 reps. That means you did the exercise 10 times in a row without any rest in between the reps.

Resistance exercise

This is a form of exercise that is meant to load the muscles by using weights in various forms. This can include free weights, Nautilus type machines, dumbbells, body weight, etc.

Sets

A set is a group of reps done in a row without resting. For example, if you are doing the bench press and you lift any given weight 8 times in a row, you are doing one set of 8 reps. After you've rested for a minute or so and you pick up the bar and do the same thing again, then you have now done two sets of 8 reps so far on the bench press.

Workout (or workout session)

This means the entire time you spent on all the sets and reps. For example, if you are doing *Pain Free Functional Strength* and are doing about 10 exercises, then the entire workout may have taken you about 45 minutes.

Chapter 1 – Have You Been Working Out Wrong?

How To Know If You've Been Working Out Wrong

Most people don't know how to workout properly. In other words they may have tried numerous times to exercise because they have heard of all the supposed benefits. But they are left disappointed and discouraged because it's not going as they had hoped. How does one know, then, if they have been working out wrong?

List of symptoms that are common for those working out wrong:

1. Excessive pain in the muscles and joints after, or even during the workout.
2. Aching joints, overall body stiffness.
3. Almost never able to function at 100% because your body is always trying to recover from previous workouts.
4. Chronic injuries – it seems every time you finally heal from one injury you get hurt again.
5. Lack of motivation – you find it harder and harder to make yourself get to the gym.
6. Perpetual pains and injuries that can go on for months, years, or even decades.
7. Prone to catch colds and other sicknesses easier than you should
8. Not getting the results you were hoping for.

Can you relate to any of the above complaints?

Then the chances are that you have not been working out properly.

What we're all looking for from our workouts:

If our workouts aren't accomplishing our goals then they need to be changed. That's where the *Pain Free Functional Strength* program comes in. After reading this book and implementing it's principals into your workout, you will be on your way to finally getting the great results you've been hoping for.

What exactly is meant by *Pain Free Functional Strength*?

Part 1. "Pain Free"

Don't all of us want to go through life pain free? Yet millions of people experience pain every day, which greatly takes away from the human experience. Obviously, all pain is not workout related, but the purpose of this book is to focus on pain that is the result of pain that is coming from improperly working out.

No Pain, No Gain?

This common saying can be heard in every gym across America, but is it true? After assisting thousands of people achieve their fitness goals, including numerous professional athletes, I can assure you that this common statement is a myth. The spirit of the saying tells us that to get good results one has to push themselves to the point of pain and beyond. Yes, for the professional athlete this does apply. But what about the majority of us who just want to look and feel our very best, those of us who simply want to check the box in knowing we're doing our part to achieve optimal health?

Will there be any pain in the *Pain Free Functional Strength* program?

It is possible that there will be some mild pain in the muscles and joints, especially in the very beginning of the workouts. As your body adapts, however, the pains disappear. After several weeks on the program you may notice that even though you are working out much harder, you're not experiencing any pain at all, either during the workout, or while your body is recovering. Imagine little to no pain associated with working out, while finally getting the great results you've always hoped for!

Part 2. "Functional Strength"

Now that the "pain free" aspect of the program has been addressed, let's take a closer look at the meaning of "functional strength". Functional strength goes way beyond it's obvious meaning. The goal of this program is to raise the quality of your life from becoming stronger as the result of your exercise program. There's nearly an infinite number of reasons to have a high level of functional strength so let's take a look at a few.

Some typical life scenarios that would benefit from having increased functional strength:
1. A mother needing to lift her young children often, or hold them in her arms
2. A broken elevator forced you to have to use the stairs and go up several floors
3. A friend bought a couch at a yard sale and asked for your help in unloading it
4. You and a friend go hunting and have to traverse several miles of tough terrain
5. The kids ask you to join them in the annual Thanksgiving day football game
6. You bought a lot more groceries than usual and you have to go up stairs to unload them
7. You get a flat tire in a remote location and have to walk a couple miles to get help

By now you get the point. There's no end to situations like those mentioned that life can throw at us at any given moment. How wonderful it is to face life's challenges knowing that your body is ready, able to perform at a high level and meet the challenge, pain free.

One last scenario, God forbid!

What if a big-time global emergency happened and you were suddenly thrust into a life or death situation? Would you be ready, with your current level of fitness? For example, what if the power grid went out and there was no electricity? With all the unrest going on in the world wouldn't it be nice to have the peace of mind knowing that you were physically ready for such an event? There's no guarantee we're all going to have it so good for our whole lifetime. Later on we'll dive into the details of the actual program. Next, let's have a look at those who can benefit from the *Pain Free Functional Strength* program.

Chapter 2 – *The Pain Free Functional Strength* Program Explained

Simply put, **Pain Free Functional Strength** is for the overwhelming majority of people who desire to look and feel their best without wanting to get hurt. But we can't spend all day in the gym. We have families, jobs, responsibilities in our places of worship, volunteer hours, a social life, etc. We want to exercise to live, not live to exercise. Sure, we want to look and feel our best, but we have no desire to spend all day in the gym. We realize that when company comes from out of town, they are now the priority; our workouts may have to take a back seat for a few days. When little Johnny catches a cold, Mom just might have to stay home with him until he gets better. We want a workout that's easy to follow, that gets us great results, and most importantly, doesn't injure us (lots more on that later). There's now no need to obsess. You no longer need to fret if life gets in the way. This is a very doable, have-a-life friendly, workout…for all of us.

A basic overview of how the *Pain Free Functional Strength* works:

The core of **Pain Free Functional Strength's** success was derived from a very basic, yet powerful, scientific principal called "repeating progressive resistance". This means adding weight slowly to match the natural progression and adaptation of your changing body.

Pain Free Functional Strength is a workout meant to be done with "resistance exercise." In other words, it's considered a "weightlifting" program. It does not include cardiovascular training (more on that later), rather it is designed to strengthen and sculpt the body with almost no risk of injury. All kinds of resistance devices work well with **Pain Free Functional Strength.** These can include:

- Free weights – straight bars, curl bars, or other assorted bars that can be loaded with any amount of weight according to your level of strength.
- Dumbbells
- Weightlifting machines such as Nautilus or Hammer Strength. These machines can work particularly well if they have a way to make the small increase needed such as adjustable pins, or small accessory weights that can be added to the main weight stack.
- Body weight exercises such as dips and chin-ups.

Here's the basics of how it works:

You will start each exercise on the light side, possibly lighter than you're used to. If you are one of the many "heavy lifting junkies", (and you know who you are – read on!) than this is going to feel too light for you, but hang in there. The first workout you will do 3 sets of 8 repetitions (the terms "sets" and "reps" are explained in detail in the glossary of terms found in the beginning of this book) on each exercise. The following workout you will do 3 sets of 9 reps on all the exercises. And again, the next workout you will do 3 sets of 10 reps, 3 sets of 11 reps the next workout and 3 sets of 12 reps the fifth workout. Here is where it changes. Once you have completed 3 sets of 12 repetitions on any given exercise, you are now ready to increase the weight for the next workout, but the reps go back down to 8. So, for the next workout you will be doing 3 sets of 8 reps per exercise, but now at the increased weight. How much heavier? Much more on that later, but for now, about a modest 5 to 10 percent increase. The next workout you will do 3 sets of 9 reps, next 3 sets of 10 reps, next workout 3 sets pf 11 reps, next 3 sets of 12 reps, then increase the weights 5 to 10 percent, reps back to 8, and repeat this formula over and over again. Eventually you will no longer be able to increase the weight and still get your reps, but this will be explained later in detail. As you go through this process of repetition, your body will continue to adapt and change rhythmically to these changing weights and rep counts. There's something very special about this simplistic methodology – I've seen nearly miraculous results for over 3 decades!

On what authority, how can you trust the *Pain Free Functional Strength program?*

Whenever I am getting ready to hire someone for a job or project, naturally I want to know what their credentials are. Do they know what they're talking about? How much experience do they have? So, what about me – how can you know and trust that I know what I'm talking about? Do I have the needed experience and successful track record to give you the confidence that I know what I'm talking about? More importantly, have the people who have hired me gotten the results they were hoping for? Please understand that I am not giving you this list of credentials for any braggadocious motivation. Rather, I want you to be able to trust me with one of your most precious possessions – your very health and well-being! So next I'm going to give you some of my experience and credentials so that you can be certain that what I'm telling you is credible, trustworthy, and accurate. Here is that list:

- Master's Degree in Exercise Physiology
- 33 years of experience helping people obtain their fitness goals
- Over 35,000 hours of one on one fitness training
- Weight loss specialist
- Weight gain expert
- Have worked with ages 8 through 80
- Have experience with almost every injury imaginable including problem areas like the lower back, shoulders, knees, hips, and many more.

- I have worked extensively with players from about half of the teams in the National Football League including the Dallas Cowboys, The Philadelphia Eagles, The Seattle Seahawks, The Kansas City Chiefs, The Miami Dolphins, The Pittsburg Steelers, to name a few.
- Clients of mine have won 7 super bowls and now proudly wear their super bowl rings
- My clients have been selected for 23 appearances in the National Football's elite – the Pro Bowl in Hawaii.
- One client of mine was on a World Series winning baseball team and I proudly held up the prestigious World Series trophy with him.
- Another client of mine won the US Open golf tournament. When he signed me an autographed photo, he wrote on it "to Mike, thank you for making me better"
- I have been in Sports Illustrated magazine, USA Today Newspaper, have been mentioned by name on Monday Night Football to name a few.
- I have flown around the country to help some of the world's greatest athletes obtain their fitness goals (translating into ridiculously large salaries!)
- My final and most important credential? I feel that God has gifted me with much wisdom and experience in the field of health, fitness and nutrition. It would be my honor to help you now, as I have those above, to let me help you look and feel your very best with the ultimate goal of improving your quality of life. I know with all the confidence that comes from this vast experience, that *Pain Free Functional Strength* will do this for you.

Next let's take a look at some categories of people who have seen great results using the *Pain Free Functional Strength program:*

1. Those who simply want to "check the box"

By this I mean those of us who want to do their part in making sure we are doing our part to obtain optimal health. You have probably heard of the endless litany of health benefits from working out, so you want to be sure you are at least doing your part to reap those rewards. Also, you want to do this as efficiently as you possibly can, not wanting to waste your valuable time.

2. Young people and those just getting started:

So lucky are you- younger person or older person- who has never worked out before, to have *Pain Free Functional Strength* as your very first workout program! *Pain Free Functional Strength* is the perfect workout for the person who is first being introduced to working out. It's a perfect fit for teens and pre-teens in high school and middle school. *Pain Free Functional Strength* should be the very first workout of every young person in school gym classes across the country. Why? Because this workout is the ideal introductory program. It takes a person from where they are at and gradually brings them along in a way that is safe, builds confidence and self-esteem and gets them the exceptional results they were hoping for.

3. Those that are fed up with getting injured from working out:

Let's revisit a basic reality check – the goal of working out is not to injure yourself! But after watching people in gyms for over 3 decades I sometimes wonder. If you're one of the millions of people who have hurt themselves while working out, there's now hope for you. There are lots of reasons you've gotten hurt in the gym, but two main ones. First, the main reason for gym injuries is simple – you tried to lift a weight that was too heavy when your body was not yet prepared. Second, your technique may have been incorrect causing your injury. But now you can proceed with working out again with almost no risk of hurting yourself in the gym ever again. This is the beauty of the *Pain Free Functional Strength* workout system. This program was designed for this reason, and to date, I have never seen a person get a single injury of any sort while doing *Pain Free Functional Strength* in over 30 years of training – now there's a track record you can trust!

4. Off Season Sports Athletes:

Pain Free Functional Strength is the perfect workout for athletes in the off season. When timed properly with your sport season, it allows your body to heal while at the same time brings on the strength increases you need for your sport. It's a beautiful thing really.

I have used this workout repeatedly on some of the best football players in the National Football League. I've listened to their complaints that the workouts were "too easy" with a big smile on my face knowing that this easier phase would be ending very soon. As their workouts did get harder, I knew that their beaten and battered bodies were now healed enough for the more strenuous lifting.

Thankful for the Results:

One of these athletes is Nate Newton, a famous offensive lineman that played with the Dallas Cowboys back in the 1990s. Under my training Nate went on to six pro bowl appearances to go along with his 3 super bowl rings. Nate will be the first to tell you how the training I gave him transformed his career.

On one occasion Nate flew me to Dallas for a game against the Philadelphia Eagles going against another client of mine – Mike Golic of the famed ESPN radio show "Mike and Mike". But a couple days before the game Nate had me over to his house. We stood in the driveway and he clicked open the garage door and said, "I want to show you what you bought me". Knowing I had never bought Nate anything, I looked into the garage with great interest. There before us was a beautiful, brand new, black Mercedes Benz convertible valued at over $200,000 in today's money. I looked at him with a puzzled look and he said "Because you've made me a much better athlete and able to play ball at a higher level than ever before, I have been financially rewarded because of it and I wanted to thank you." How deeply moved with appreciation I was at this gesture of thankfulness.

5.   The non-athletic type:

Do you consider yourself the non-athlete type? Maybe you're a little uncoordinated and it feels unnatural when you've tried working out in the past. Perhaps you felt awkward and out of place. You may have even been among those who were chosen last as a kid when sports teams were being decided. Fear not! Please give *Pain Free Functional Strength* a try – it's the perfect workout for you! I have seen nearly miraculous transformations over the years of people who thought they weren't the workout type.

Meet Alex

Years ago, I had a client who fit this category exactly. He had never been the athletic type but was desperate to shape up his out of tone body. When he hired me, he sheepishly asked "Do you really think I can do this?" I quickly replied, "I don't think you can do it; I know you can!" At first Alex struggled under even the lightest weights. But because of the power of the science behind *Pain Free Functional Strength,* within a couple months Alex had made amazing strides and was even getting some turned heads in the gym. "What is that guy doing? He's really showing results!"

It was so deeply embedded in Alex's head that he wasn't the athletic type that he was scared to death to do the bench press using those large, intimidating 45 pound plates, even though he had now built up to that level. So, I had to use smaller plates to add up to the larger amount just to keep him at ease.

Alex definitely fit the non-athlete profile when we started. But within a year, he developed quite the nice athletic physique and was able to bench press nearly 200 pounds, even though he only weighed about 170 pounds. He could now feel proud wearing a tank top and other athletic apparel. Alex needed *Pain Free Functional Strength.* It transformed his life, and it can transform yours.

6.   Those coming off an injury, rehab, or physical therapy:

Pain Free Functional Strength is the perfect workout as a follow up for those who have finished with these situations. People coming off injuries are usually feeling flabby and out of shape and are anxious to get back to working out. But there is sometimes an underlying fear that a re-injury might occur. If you don't make a smart comeback then that re-injury thought could become reality. Re-injuring a partially healed or completely healed area of the body can be a true anatomical disaster. Why? Because if the trouble spot is freshly re-injured, you have a much greater chance of it bothering you for the rest of your life. Please don't ignore this nugget of wisdom I've gleaned from so many hours in the gym. If you ignore it, you may have the rest of your life to wish you hadn't. Make your comeback deliberately slow, methodical, and smart. *Pain Free Functional Strength* is the perfect workout to bring you back to shape.

Matt's story

"I was doing bicep curls as heavy as I could, doing a few sets of only 3 or 4 reps" explained Matt, a very advanced body builder. Matt continued. "When my bicep tendon snapped, it was so loud that everyone in the gym stopped what they were doing in unison to find the source of that awful sound." I cringed at the finale of the story and the damage to his bicep was obvious. His left bicep muscle had atrophied (shrunk) to a paltry size compared to his other arm, which boasted a large, robust upper arm.

But Matt was determined to get it right this time and for the next several months we carefully navigated his way through a lengthy round of *Pain Free Functional Strength*. After several months Matt's injured left arm was nearly as large as the other. This is another true to life success story attributed to *Pain Free Functional Strength.*

7.   The overweight:

Yes, *Pain Free Functional Strength* is the perfect workout if losing weight is your goal. And ladies, don't worry. This is not a "bulk you up" workout! I have witnessed countless times overweight people losing weight and toning up using this superior workout. But I must warn you in advance. *Pain Free Functional Strength* is not a quick fix to weight loss. Rather, it fits into a solid, long term strategy for obtaining and keeping long term results. There are several reasons why *Pain Free Functional Strength* is so effective for weight loss, but the nature of the program is a good fit for those wanting to shed unwanted fat. Because the workout is so specific and easy to follow, they are much more likely to stick with it for the long haul. Within weeks, people who struggle with their weight can see tangible, visible results. Areas that were sagging are now starting to lift. Spots that had no tone at all are now emerging into more clearly defined muscles. Once these changes are noticed, exercisers get excited and work even harder at their diets and cardio training to complement their *Pain Free Functional Strength* workouts.

Joe's Story

My phone rang and on the other end was the general manager of one of the teams from the National Football League. He told me of a player that was really struggling with his weight and he needed some help. It was springtime, and that's when a lot of NFL players panic knowing spring training is right around the corner. I told him to send Joe down and we'd see what I could do.

When I met Joe, I was amazed at his size, even though I worked with a lot of guys from the NFL. He stood 6 feet, 8 inches tall and weighed well over 400 pounds. I put him on a strict diet, and we did lots of bike riding for his cardio. For his gym workout I prescribed, you guessed it, *Pain Free Functional Strength.* After only 4 weeks Joe was thrilled to see a loss of over 40 pounds – more than a pound per day! Of course, *Pain Free Functional Strength* wasn't the only factor in his success, but it was an important piece of the weight loss puzzle.

8.   Baby boomers

If you're in that 50 something age group and older, look no further for the perfect, tailor made workout program. How do I know this? Because I am proudly one of you! I do *Pain Free Functional Strength* myself now as my go to work out. I love the way it starts out easier, then slowly, week by week, builds me up to the heavier weeks. And as an older guy, I love when I get to the more difficult weeks so I can prove to myself "I still got it!". That's important to us older guys. But seriously, this is a great workout for this age group, both male and female. Give it a try and see for yourself.

In Summary

Just about everyone can benefit from ***Pain Free Functional Strength.*** From the elite athlete to the non-athletic type to those coming off injuries, or those wanting to lose weight, ***Pain Free Functional Strength*** will amaze you at the results you can get.

Mary's Story

Mary was a single woman in her early 20's who was on a mission when she hired me to take her to the next level with her health and fitness. Like so many, she wanted to look and feel her very best but had little idea of how to go about it. After all, look at all the conflicting advice out there now. I started Mary on ***Pain Free Functional Strength*** right away and advised her on how to eat properly and how to go about her cardiovascular exercise. Mary was highly motivated and did everything I told her to the letter. She worked very hard in the months that followed, putting it all together like a well-tuned orchestra.

Something wonderful happened to Mary during this time in her life. Naturally her body responded, and she went from having a decent figure for a young woman to being truly stunning. Instead of slumping, Mary now stood erect. She walked with confidence and had a different spirit about her. Her skin tone was radiant, and she took on a healthy glow. She was confident, felt much better about herself, and sculpted a beautiful and healthy feminine physique.

One workout Mary showed up with a big smile and greeted me with an unusual big hug. She was thrilled to share her success story with me. Mary was chosen for employee of the year out of over 100 other employees. She told me that all these workouts had paid off for her in big dividends, both in the way she felt, and financially. Did Mary win employee of the year just because of her working out? Probably not, but I'm sure she would be the first to tell you that it was a large part of her success.

Chapter 3 – The Great Mistake

In the world of observing fitness and working out, I have a great advantage over many others. This advantage is that I have been able to carefully observe for over 35,000 hours, what people do in gyms to get in shape. Early on in my career, back in the early 1980's, something troubling started to come into focus. Over the decades this observation strengthened and crystallized into something I now call "the great mistake". What is the great mistake? It's when people push themselves to the limit or are pushed to the limits by a partner or trainer, long before they can handle it.

A Parking Lot Encounter

I was working at a large gym as a personal trainer long before it became in vogue. In fact, there was only 2 of us fitness trainers despite the gym boasting a membership of over 5,000. As I was leaving a fitness session walking to my car, a middle-aged woman stopped me with a desperate look on her face and said, "Can I please have one of your business cards?" "Sure" I said, as I handed her the card. She went on to say "I am furious with that other trainer. He worked me out so hard on the first visit that I could not walk for two days!"

I never heard from her again. I am guessing that she was so angered and upset over this ridiculous and dangerous treatment that she never came back, or worse, completely gave up on the thought of working out.

A Real-Life Heavy Weights Junkie

I'll never forget Bill, a man in his early 30's who was truly addicted to lifting excessively heavy weights – even though he knew he was hurting himself! People in the gym would cringe watching Bill work out. He wore loose bulky clothes which covered his stocky, but very mediocre body. We would watch him load the bar on exercises like squats, the bench press, and deadlifts, piling on 45-pound plate after plate obtaining final counts well in excess of 500 pounds. He would recruit a couple young guys in the gym to spot him as he would go through his ritual. On each lift, his face would turn beet red and I can remember vividly the veins popping out of his face and neck. After doing a few reps and banging the weights back down to the floor with poor control, he would rest 5 to 10 minutes before doing the next set.

I spoke with Bill one day candidly about his workouts and was shocked at our dialogue. He confessed that every morning he would get out of bed with great pain for several minutes until his body finally got mobile enough to move around. He knew that what he was doing was more harmful than good but there was something about the rush of mastering the heavy weights that kept bringing him back to the gym for this self-imposed punishment. If all this work and time paid dividends for great physical, and or mental well-being, one could at least understand going through such pain. But it did exactly the opposite. Because of his addiction to heavy weights Bill was literally ruining his young body I knew that if he didn't stop this behavior, the forecast for his later years would be very painful and bleak.

I realize that there are not many exercisers that take things to this extreme. But this true story is included to make sure that you can learn a lesson from Bill. If you're going to spend time in the gym, make sure that what you're doing is for your good, to help you achieve your goal of looking and feeling your best, and being in great health. Following the *Pain Free Functional Strength* workout program will ensure exactly that.

Working Out and Fertilizer Have This in Common

An under confident trainer can be a deadly combination. Because of their lack of knowledge or experience as a trainer, they will often brutalize the poor, unsuspecting client who is ill prepared for such an assault. I've seen this play out numerous times in gyms. People come away from these encounters either injured or discouraged to the point of quitting altogether.

So, what does fertilizer have to do with all this? Working out with weights and fertilizer have something particularly important in common. The user must know just the right amount to apply for best results. If too little fertilizer is used than the plants will not grow to their potential. If you apply too much than you can damage, or even kill the plants. It's the same thing with working out. Not lifting heavy enough will bring slow progress. Lifting too heavy will result in injury sooner or later. The good trainer will know just how much "fertilizer" to apply to their client. This conscientious trainer wants his or her client to get great results, without the risk of injury.

The Great Mistake Antidote

Pain Free Functional Strength is the antidote to the "great mistake". If you follow this tried and proven program, you can be assured that you are applying just the right amount of "fertilizer" to produce long lasting results for looking and feeling your absolute best.

It's Time for a Paradigm Shift in the Way it's Always Been Done

Please read the following scenario carefully – it plays out across America in schools and gyms across the country thousands of times each year. I call it "the caveman approach to weightlifting". What happens is a group of people get together in a gym, this is especially true of teens and preteens, under the care of an instructor or not, and a sort of survival of the fittest ritual breaks out. "How much can you bench press Billy?" or "oh c'mon, you can do more weight than that!" Without proper instruction, kids especially gravitate to this Neanderthal way of doing things, desperately trying to prove themselves by lifting heavy weights in front of the instructor or their peers. With nearly 100 percent consistency, a couple of the kids will really shine and be able to lift heavy weights and be the heroes. These chosen few were almost certainly genetically gifted to be able to lift heavier that their peers. It probably had little or nothing to do with any prior superior training; it was most certainly all in the genes. In many cases it's also the kids who simply reached puberty earlier.

Please don't misunderstand me, there are many who have used the caveman approach and gotten good results. Many people do work out very hard most of time and look great. What I am saying is that for most people, this is a poor long-term strategy that almost guarantees injury, unnecessary chronic soreness, and stiffness, and ultimately, quitting working out altogether. Do you remember the story of the turtle and the hare? If you're a hare, somewhere down the road you can expect to be passed by this happy, healthy, pain free turtle.

The Rest of Us

But what about the other 90 percent of the classmates, the ones who performed at a more mere-mortal level? In other words, what happened to the "rest of us"? This is the sad part. Many will conclude "well I guess working out isn't for me" or even worse, "I guess this is just another thing I'm no good at". There's the crime! Put any kid on a superior weightlifting program like *Pain Free Functional Strength,* no matter how skinny or overweight they are and watch their beautiful youthful bodies change for the better! And as a side bonus they are learning a great lesson for life – hard work and patience pay dividends for long term success, there are no quick fixes!

A Recent Court Case

A while ago, I was hired by attorneys for a jury trial as an expert witness for a young teen-aged boy. He was a victim of this ridiculous cave man approach that was mentioned earlier. The instructor had each student try to lift as heavy as they could using a leg press machine for just a few repetitions. Skinny young boys faced with the fear of looking weak in front of their peers will just about kill themselves to lift heavy enough to save face. When pushing with all his might with the class and instructor looking on, he felt a sharp pain in his lower back. His outcome was not good. Now in his 20's, he has a permanent, persistent back problem that has robbed him of the joy of a normal healthy life. If only this poor young man would have had a scientifically grounded workout like *Pain Free Functional Strength* to start with, his tragic outcome would have never happened.

In Conclusion

Our society is long overdue to replace this ridiculous cave man approach in gyms to a new age of enlightenment and reason. It's high time to take off the animal skins and put down the clubs and spears and put on the garment of knowledge and modern scientific advancement. We can now all finally agree that there is too much insanity woven into the way we're doing it now, and frankly, it's not working for the majority of people. This inferior methodology has as its offspring injury, discouragement, and quitting altogether. It's time to get it right with a proper program that delivers great results with almost no risk of injury – *Pain Free Functional Strength.*

Chapter 4 – Mentally Preparing Ahead for Pain *Free Functional Strength*

Before Starting

We are almost ready to get on the program but entering it with the proper mindset is critically important. In other words, the more mentally prepared we are ahead of time, the greater the chance we will have positive long-term results. But there are some real pit falls out there that can shipwreck even the most determined fitness enthusiasts. I don't want this to happen to you. I want you to look and feel your best without getting hurt. So, study the following mental preparations carefully. These guidelines will help you stay on course even when the going gets rough.

Mental Prep #1 - Pick a Time Period That Will Allow You to Focus

It's very discouraging to start a fitness program only to be derailed over and over again. Some of you know exactly what I'm talking about. If you're like most, there will never be a time that is absolutely perfect. Life just doesn't seem to work that way. But there are times that are better than others. Look at you schedule. Only you can figure out a good time period to get started. After the holidays usually works well, or when the kids return to school in the fall is often another good time to start. Is there a major life event on the horizon that might be too distracting?

Examples of Major Events That Could Sabotage A Fitness Program:

* a job change
* getting ready to move or just having moved in
* high school or college end of semester exams
* preparing for a wedding
* going through a divorce
* just had a baby
* busy time at work

On the other hand, once you've done *Pain Free Functional Strength* a couple times and are familiar with how it works, you will find it easier to fit it in during just about any of life's challenges. But if it's your first time you have a better chance of success if you pick a time period of at least 4 weeks where you can focus your attention on the program.

Mental Prep #2 – Have Realistic Expectations

So, you've decided to give *Pain Free Functional Strength* a try because you definitely want to look and feel your best with almost zero risk of getting hurt - wise decision. But what can you expect in the way of results, and how long will it take? These are valid questions most participants want to know up front. It's important that you realize right from the start that *Pain Free Functional Strength* is not a quick fix. For over 30 years I've been carefully keeping my antennae up, watching and waiting for that magic bullet, that pill giving instant results, or any other fast track to a lean, beautiful body. Let's all just agree together and move forward – there is no such thing and most likely there never will!

It takes time:

It will take several weeks using *Pain Free Functional Strength* to see or feel any significant difference. That's because *Pain Free Functional Strength* is more of a solid, long term strategy rather than a quick fix. The first few weeks you are not struggling under excessively heavy weights. Rather you are concentrating on good from on each exercise as you gradually make the scheduled increases on your weights and reps. It is during this critical first phase that changes are taking place internally that will set the stage for getting great visible results later.

After 3-4 months on *Pain Free Functional Strength,* you should see and feel amazing changes both in your appearance and in the way you feel. Along with the obvious physical changes there will be side bonuses of increased self-confidence and a raised ability to deal with life's many challenges. You will have gained muscle tone while decreasing unwanted fat. Clothes will fit better, or you may even need to start replacing your wardrobe.

Mental Prep #3 – Understand in Advance the 3 Phases of Pain Free Functional Strength

When you go through a cycle of *Pain Free Functional Strength* there are 3 levels that you will be journeying through. These are 1.) The easier phase, 2.) The moderate phase and 3.) The difficult phase, oftentimes referred to as "the results phase". It's important that you understand and accept the wisdom of the program. So if, for example, you are in the easy phase and are getting impatient and want to bump up your weights ahead of schedule, you will refrain from doing so because you know it's wiser in the long run to just follow the program.

Also, know that there is no official beginning or end to the 3 phases of Pain Free Functional Strength: it's all very subjective.

A Recap of What to Expect During Phase 1, 2 and 3 While on *Pain Free Functional Strength*

Phase 1 – The light phase.

During this phase the weights should be on the light side. You are getting familiar with the exercises and working on making sure your form is correct. This is also the phase in which you will "even it out" after the second week to balance out the 8,9,10,11, and 12 rep count to be about equal. Phase 1 can last from 3 or 4 weeks up to about 5 or 6 weeks if you started the program on the lighter side (perfectly fine when doing *Pain Free Functional Strength.)*

Phase 2 – The transition phase.

During phase 2 you will be transitioning to the much harder phase 3. Now the weights are getting harder, but each exercise you are able to get the prescribed number of sets and reps without too much of a struggle. As with the other phases, there is no official beginning or end to phase 2; it's all very subjective. This phase could last from about 3 to 5 weeks.

Phase 3 – The difficult phase, commonly called the "results phase".

At this point in the workout, the weights have gotten heavy. During phase 3, your will mind will often drift ahead to the upcoming workouts with thoughts like "how on earth am I going to get my 12's, I'm struggling to get my 8's!" This is very normal, but keep in mind that it's during phase 3 that you will be reaping most of the benefits of the entire *Pain Free Functional Strength* workout. Don't preoccupy your mind with future workouts; focus on each exercise and workout as they come. Challenge yourself. Just how far can you take an exercise before it finally comes to an end? During phase 3 you will actually feel yourself getting stronger and stronger, from workout to workout. This most difficult phase can last for about 2 to 6 weeks for most. But again, if it's more or less for you that's OK, this built-in flexibility is one of the beauties of this program. It's also during phase 3 that each exercise will come to an end (after going 2 workouts in a row where you cannot get the prescribed number of reps) and you will be deciding what to do next.

You must discipline yourself!

As you progress through *Pain Free Functional Strength* keep in mind the 3 general phases and discipline yourself to stay on the plan. In the first easier phase (from the start to about week 4), you are concentrating on good form as you settle into the program. Lifting should not be too hard, just yet. In the second phase (about weeks 5 through 8), things are getting tougher now. You are still able to do the prescribed numbers of sets and reps but it's not going as easy, like in the first few weeks. Finally comes the difficult phase (approximately weeks 9 through 12). During this phase it's now gotten down-right hard to get the prescribed numbers of sets and reps. But no need to worry. The first 2 phases have prepared you and your body is now ready for the challenge.

The number of weeks for each phase is not exact:

Be aware that the above time frames for each phase are not exact; this greatly depends on how you set the weights in the beginning. A few weeks more or less on any of the phases is absolutely OK. It's not uncommon for people to go as long as six months on the same *Pain Free Functional Strength* cycle, progressing with great care and precision, and getting fabulous results.

The official end of an exercise on Pain Free Functional Strength:

When you go 2 workouts in a row and are not able to do the number of reps that the program called for on any given exercise, you have finished *Pain Free Functional Strength,* (for that exercise – much more on this later)

Now do you understand the big picture of *Pain Free Functional Strength?* It is important that you get this before actually starting on the program.

Mental Prep # 4 – Be Prepared Ahead of Time for Life's Challenges

If you ever want to prove to yourself what an imperfect world we live in, start a great program like *Pain Free Functional Strength* and watch for all the difficulties to pop up, trying to derail you from your efforts. I'm talking about life here, and *Pain Free Functional Strength* is the ideal workout for the rest of us, which was designed just for this - to get the results we want despite life's many challenges. Don't let this discourage you, rather, be mentally ready for it in advance.

Life's Challenges:

What kind of challenges am I talking about? You know the ones. You're 2 or 3 weeks into the program and feeling really good about it, and then you get sick. Or you're happy you've made it into phase 2 and your boss gives you a big project with an unrealistic deadline. One more example (out of the thousands!), your daughter's softball team did surprisingly well and they now have a couple weeks of travel for playoff games – and you were really looking great after a couple months on *Pain Free Functional Strength!*

There's No Longer Any Need to Quit:

You no longer have to worry about failing when struck with life's challenges while you're on Pain Free Functional Strength. Remember, this program is a workout for the rest of us. We have a life. Things happen that are out of our control. In fact, the program was designed with this in mind! There are strategies built into *Pain Free Functional Strength* to enable you to jump these hurdles with ease. For example, if you miss a week due to illness, when you return you can simply lower the weights down a notch or two to where it feels like it did when you had to stop. Or you may be surprised to discover that you were able to start right back where you left off. *Pain Free Functional Strength* was designed to be flexible, to allow for, and even anticipate, marching forward despite life's predictable unpredictability.

Mental Prep # 5 – Have a Goal or Something to Shoot For

A wonderful bonus of *Pain Free Functional Strength* is that it's a self-motivating program. Once you understand it and are going through the prescribed sets and reps, the program can draw you in. It's not uncommon for people on *Pain Free Functional Strength* to anxiously anticipate their next workout, how it will feel, how well they will do not?

Here's another idea for your consideration. Have a concrete goal in mind before starting *Pain Free Functional Strength.* In other words, you may want to try and tie the program into a motivating long-term goal, several weeks, or even months into the future. Your plan of action could sound like this: "When I have finished this round of *Pain Free Functional Strength,* I want to run a 5 K road race", and then even pre-register for the event.

Here Are a Few More Examples of Goal Setting Based Around the *Pain Free Functional Strength* System

* When I finish *Pain Free Functional Strength* I will reward myself with a cruise
* I want to look my best for my wedding next year so I will do at least 2 rounds of *Pain Free Functional Strength*
* I am going to try to lose 20 pounds during this round of *Pain Free Functional Strength*
* My class reunion is in 4 months. I really want to look good for it.
* Football season starts in 6 months. I will do at least 2 rounds of *Pain Free Functional Strength* to heal and strengthen myself to be ready.
* I will be interviewing for jobs in 3 months so I will finish a round of *Pain Free Functional Strength* so I can look good and feel confident.

What goal or dream do you have that you want to be ready for? Consider these goals and then come up with a few of your own to tie into your own personal *Pain Free Functional Strength* workout.

Mental Prep # 6 – Keep in Mind the Hundreds of Benefits as a Result of *Pain Free Functional Strength*

It's very easy to get caught up in the physical, visible improvements when doing Pain Free Functional Strength. But what's going on under the skin? This is the real miracle when it comes to exercise. I have witnessed true transformations in thousands of people. The following is a very small list of the benefits that will be taking place as you proceed through *Pain Free Functional Strength,* most of these happen "behind the scenes". In other words, there are very real benefits that happen which can't necessarily be seen or detected.

Psychological Benefits

- More self-confidence
- Higher self-esteem
- Able to handle stress better
- Better moods most of the time
- You can think more clearly
- Reduced anxiety
- Sharpen memory and brain power
- Can enjoy those kids and grandkids with greater joy and energy

Physical Benefits

- Stronger Muscles – able to perform life's many tasks easier
- Stronger tendons, ligaments, and bones.
- Physically more prepared for life's many challenges
- Strengthening of the lungs, heart, and vascular system
- Reduced risk of cancer
- Reduction of unwanted fat
- Increased resistance to colds, the flu, etc.
- Increased metabolism which burns more calories even at rest
- Decreased risk of Diabetes
- Able to perform more work and with less effort
- Exercise boosts energy
- Exercise promotes better sleep
- Exercise can improve sexual drive and stamina
- Increase chances of living longer

Hopefully, you now have a good understanding of what your mindset needs to be before even starting the actual program. The next steps will deal with getting ready for the actual workout.

Chapter 5 – How to Make Small Weight Increases

Before getting to the actual workout, there are 2 more topics that need to be covered; you must get these right. The first is knowing how to increase the weights when on *Pain Free Functional Strength,* the other deals with how to choose exercises.

1. Know How to Increase Your Weights on Pain Free Functional Strength

Being able to raise your weights in small increments is a crucial part of Pain Free Functional Strength, especially when the weight is less than 50 pounds. Unfortunately, very few gyms are equipped for these small increases. Let me give you an example of what I mean. Let's assume you're a young girl and you've never worked out before. One of the exercises you decided to do is the dumbbell bicep curl. You start out using the 5-pound dumbbells and you successfully go through the 8,9,10,11, and 12 reps for your first 3 workouts. Now it's time to increase the weight and go back to 8 reps. But you notice the next smallest size is the 10-pound dumbbells, and then 15, 20 and so on. This will not work on the Pain Free Functional Strength system – the increases are way too big! When using less than 10 pounds, it's fine if the increases are not in that 5 to 10 percent range previously stated. With that said, it would be ideal to go up by one-pound increases, from 5 to 6 pounds, 6 to 7, 7 to 8 and so on.

The Solution – 3 Options for Making the Needed Small Weight Increases

Let's now look at how to make the small increases needed on each of the 3 main categories of gym apparatus –

1. Dumbbells
2. Straight bars and curl bars
3. Exercise machines

1. Dumbbells (3 choices for small weight increases)

There are hundreds of exercises that can be done with dumbbells. That's why they are such a popular choice for the *Pain Free Functional Strength* workout. As stated earlier, however, it can be very difficult to make the small increases needed using dumbbells when on *Pain Free Functional Strength*.

A. The first choice When Using Dumbbells – "Plate Mates" Magnetic Add-on Weights.

This is a name brand easily found online at sites like Amazon or eBay, or you can call them at 877-336-7483. These are magnetic add on weights that you simply stick on to your dumbbell magnetically. They come in pairs of 5/8s pound and 1 ¼ pound increments. When it is time to increase, you would make your increase from 10 pounds, for example, to 11 ¼ pounds by using the two 5/8s pound magnetic weights. The next increase you would remove the 5/8s pound weights and put on the two 1 ¼ pound weights making the dumbbells now 12 ½ pounds. You will need 2 pairs of each size if wanting to do both dumbbells at the same time.

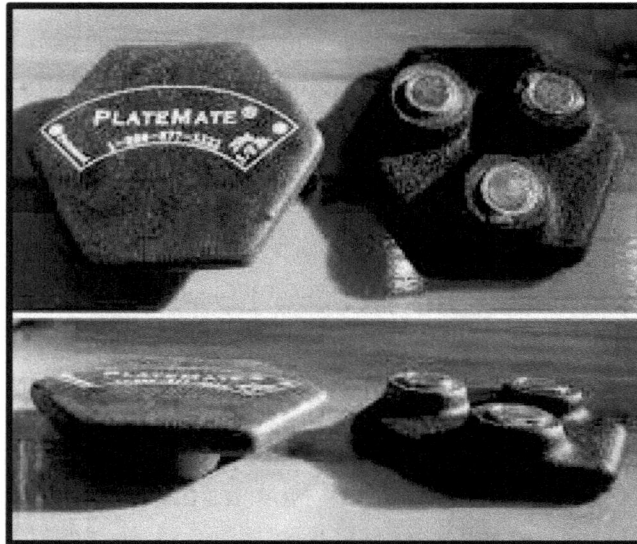

Plate Mates Magnetic add on weights allow
you to make small increases without having
to buy excessive dumbbells

This is probably the best option when making the small increases needed, but the dumbbells you are using must be made of some form of steel so that the magnets will stick. Many gyms have rubberized coated steel weights that may or may not allow for the use of these magnetic add on weights. You will simply have to try it out to see. You could easily put these in your gym bag and take them to and from the gym. Or gym owners should consider having these on hand.

B. The Second Choice When Using Dumbbells – Weighted Wrist Bands

This choice is a little cumbersome, but it does work. Here the exerciser uses weighted wrist bands to make the small increases. You can get 2 sizes, the one pound and the 2 ½ pound wrist weights, or it also works to get 3 or 4 sets of the 1-pound wrist weights. These are not as large and awkward as the larger 2 ½ pound wrist weights. So, for example, if the exercise was going to increase from 5 pounds, you could easily increase from 5 to 6 pounds by putting a one-pound wrist weight on each wrist. Next, you could go from 6 pounds to 7 ½ by using a 2 ½ pound wrist weight and on to 8 ½ using both. From there you would increase to the 10-pound dumbbell and then start the process over again. (See photos of these increases below)

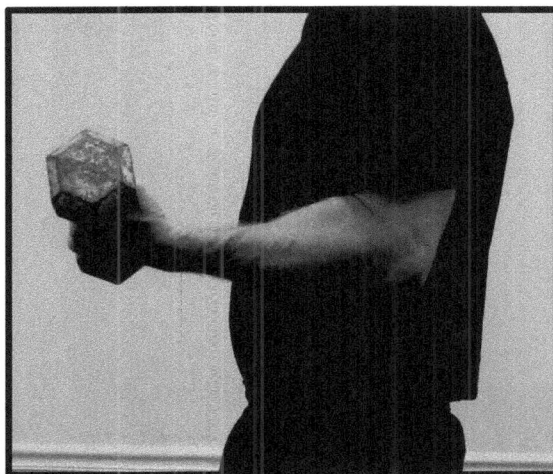

This exerciser is using a 10-pound dumbbell. After getting his 3 sets of 12 reps he will increase by 1-pound

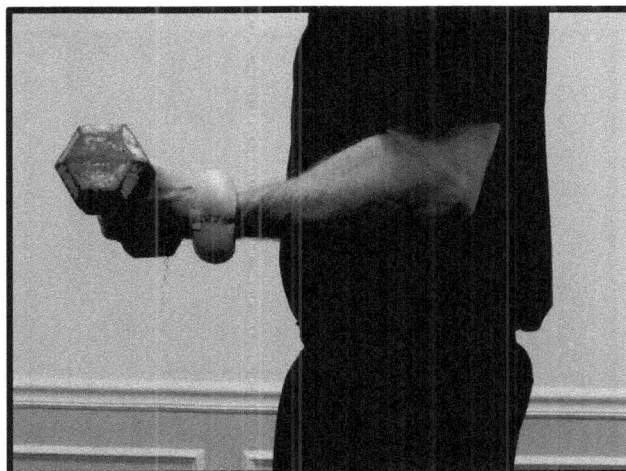

By using a one-pound wrist weight, this exerciser can go from 10 to 11-pounds.

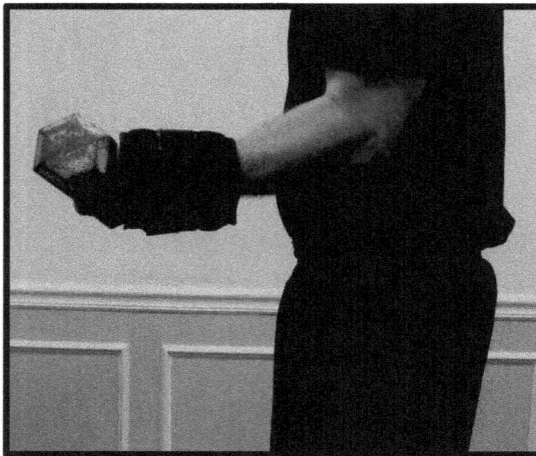

For the next weight increase the one-pound
wrist band is removed and a 2 ½-pound
wrist weight is added to make the total 12
½-pounds.

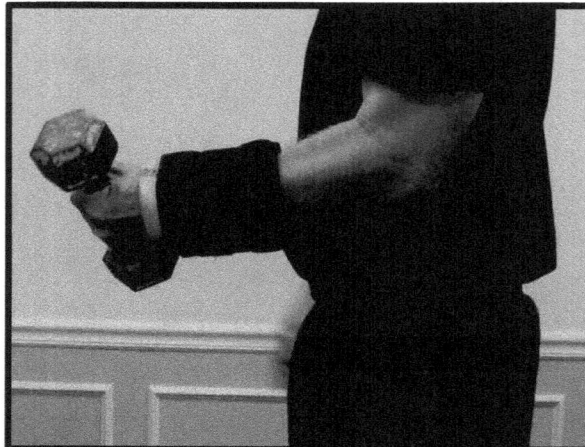

Next, along with the 2 ½-pound wrist
weight the one-pound wrist weight is added
as well, making a total of 13 ½-pounds. For
the next increase, this person would take
each wrist weights off and go to the 15-
pound dumbbells.

C. **The Third Choice When Using Dumbbells -Power Blocks (not shown)**

Power blocks are a form of dumbbell that uses an adjustment pin or dial on a stack of dumbbells that allows the user to easily change the weights in small 2- or 3-pound increments. This is an excellent choice for the person wanting to work out in a home gym because you would not have to buy several sets of dumbbells of varying sizes.

This concludes the section of making small weight increases with dumbbells. Now let's take a look at how to make these increases with the bar.

2. Bars – Both Large Straight Bars and Smaller Curl Bars (standard 2-inch diameter ends)

The Straight Bar - First let's look at the large standard sized 45-pound bar that is one of the most common items found in any gym. Because of its large size, the exerciser can simply use the 2 ½ pound plates to increase by 5 to 10 percent. (See photo)

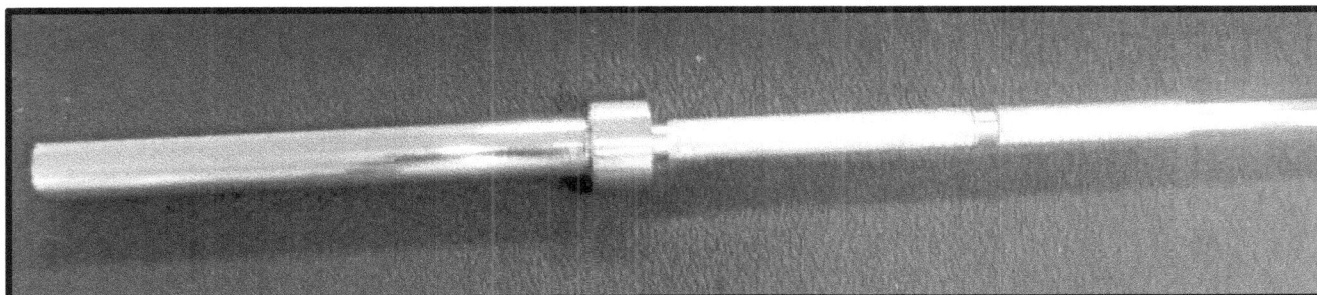

The very popular standard sized straight bar found in almost all gyms (one side shown). These bars weigh 45 pounds by themselves.

The Curl Bar – 3 Options for Small Increases.

Because curl bars weigh a lot less than the larger straight bars, about 15 pounds, the exerciser needs to get a bit more creative to make the small increases.

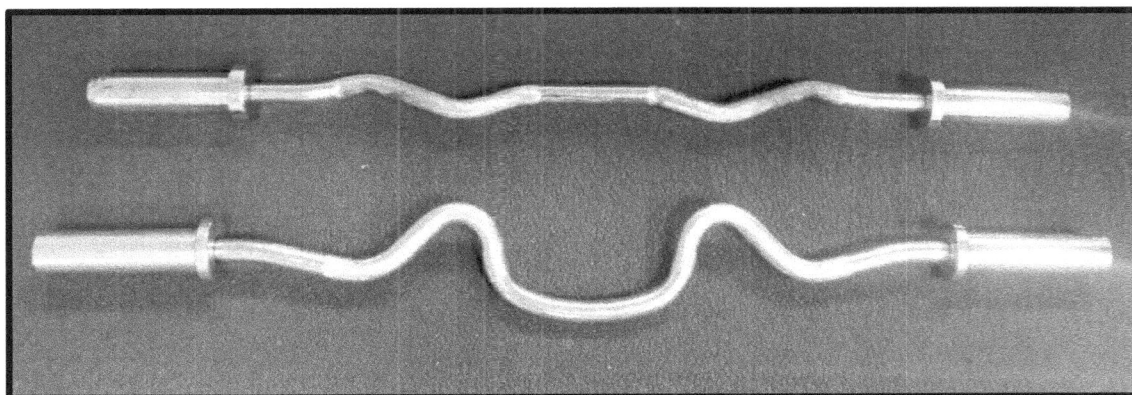

Here are 2 types of curl bars. They weigh about 15 pounds each by themselves.

Option Number One for the Curl Bar: Plate Mates

The first option is once again from the company Plate Mates. This is a great choice because they have the perfect solution – plates that weigh only 1 ¼ pounds. These also can be found online and would be the perfect solution when using the curl bar. Using the Plate Mates, the exerciser could start with the bar by itself for a weight of 15 pounds. For their first increase they could add the 1 ¼ pound Plate Mates to each side of the bar to go from 15 pounds to 17 ½ pounds. From there they would increase by removing the Plate Mates 1 ¼ pound plates and putting on the 2 ½ pound plates found in all gyms, making the weight 20 pounds.

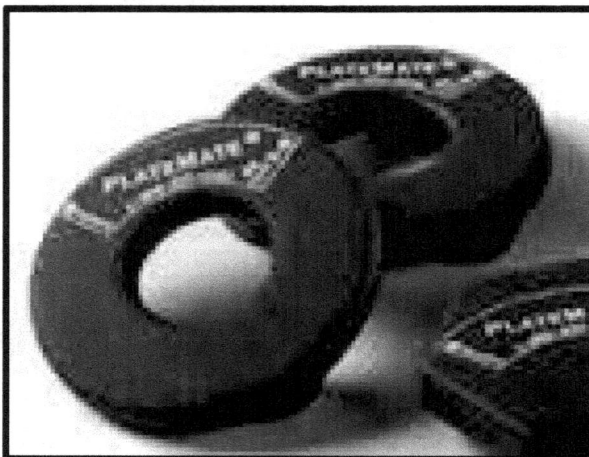

Plate Mates 1 ¼ pound plates are great for
making small increases while doing your
Pain Free Functional Strength workouts.

Option Number Two for the Curl Bar: Ader Micro Load Plates

The second option is very similar to the above Plate Mates, but it is from a different company. These are called Ader Micro-load weights, and this is the perfect choice for someone wanting to make very small increases each time. The plates come in weights of ¼ pound, ½ pound, ¾ pound, and 1 pound. It's easy to see how precise you could be using these very small plates.

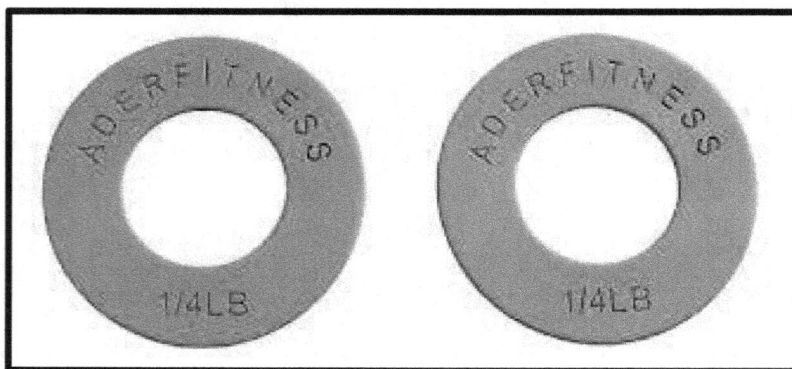

These are the Ader Fitness ¼ pound plates.
They have a wide variety of sizes perfect for
the Pain Free Functional Strength workout

Option Number Three for the Curl Bar: One Pound Compression Ring Collars

The third option uses a collar that weighs about 1 pound, or 1 ¼ pounds depending on the brand you get. These are normally referred to as pressure ring collars and they have a small handle that loosens or tightens the ring on the bar. The very popular brand Ivanko sells a pair of these that weigh 1 ¼ pounds. Since these collars weigh about a pound, they can be used to make the needed small weight increases. By using the collars on each end of the bar, the exerciser can go from 15 pounds, to 17 pounds. When it is time for the next increase, the pressure ring collars would come off and the 2 ½ pound plates would be used with the "weightless" spring collars. By using combinations of the pressure ring collars, the spring collars and the 2 ½ pound plates, the exerciser can keep the necessary small increases in weight. (See photos)

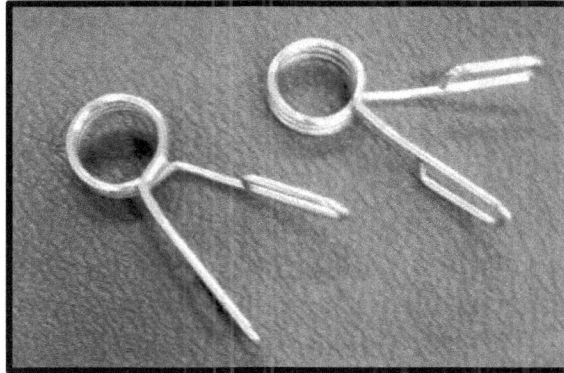

Spring collars for a 2-inch bar. These are considered having no weight.

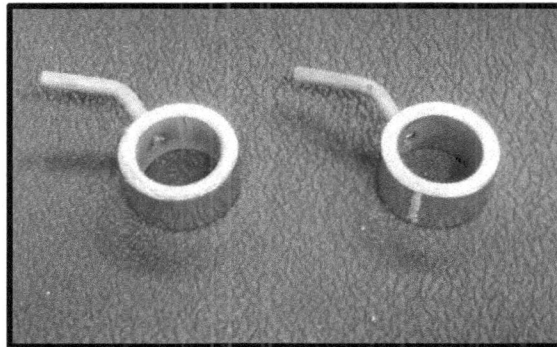

These are called compression collars and can be used as one-pound weights.

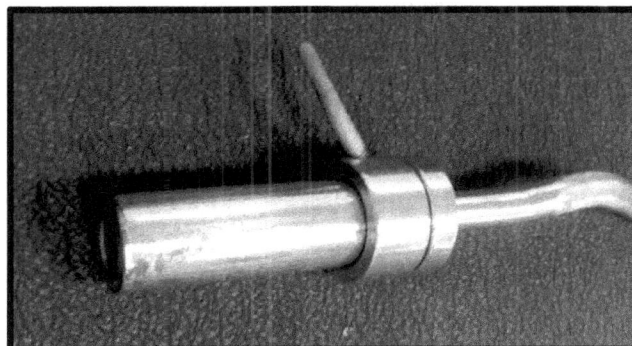

This photo shows the standard curl bar with a one-pound collar. 2 of these will make the 15-pound bar now weigh 17 pounds.

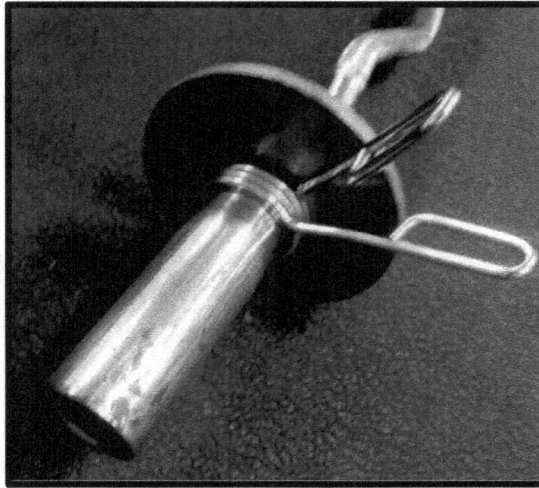

For the next weight increase the one-pound collar is removed and a 2 ½ pound plate is put on along with the spring collars making a total weight of 20 pounds.

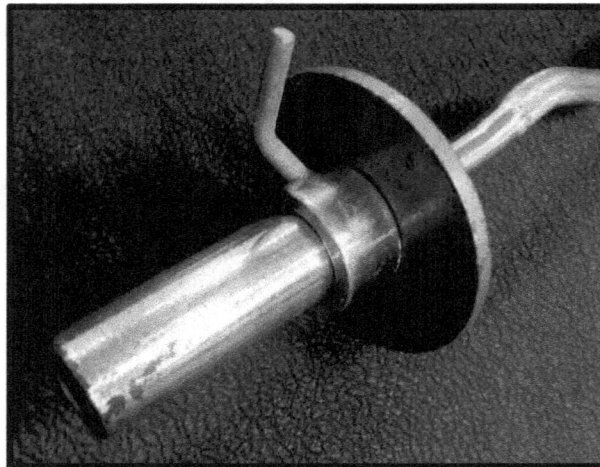

For the next weight increase we take off the spring collars and add the 1-pound collars. The total weight is now 22 pounds.

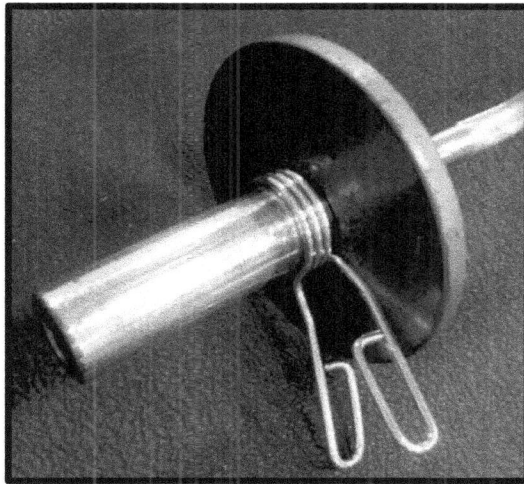

Next, the one-pound collars and the 2 ½
pound plates are removed and the next
weight increase is the 5-pound plate, making
the total weight now 25 pounds.

3. Machines – Weight Stack Type

There is a wide variety of exercise machines that have a weight stack that the exerciser uses a pin to adjust the weight, and these can be an excellent choice for the person wanting to do the *Pain Free Functional Strength* workout. As with the other choices, you just need to make sure that you can make the needed small increases. If you have to make a small increase and the machine only allows you to increase one full plate, then this machine may not be an option.

The New Machines Work Great for Pain Free Functional Strength

A wonderful new development has taken place over the past few years that has been a real breakthrough when using the *Pain Free Functional Strength* system. The Life Fitness Company, for example, has come out with a knob adjustment pin that has 4 settings. Each of these divides one plate so the user can add 5, 10 and 15 pounds to whatever weight they set. So now by simply turning the adjustment knob, you can increase from 30 to 35, 40, 45, etc. It's easy to see how perfect these machines are for the *Pain Free Functional Strength* workouts.

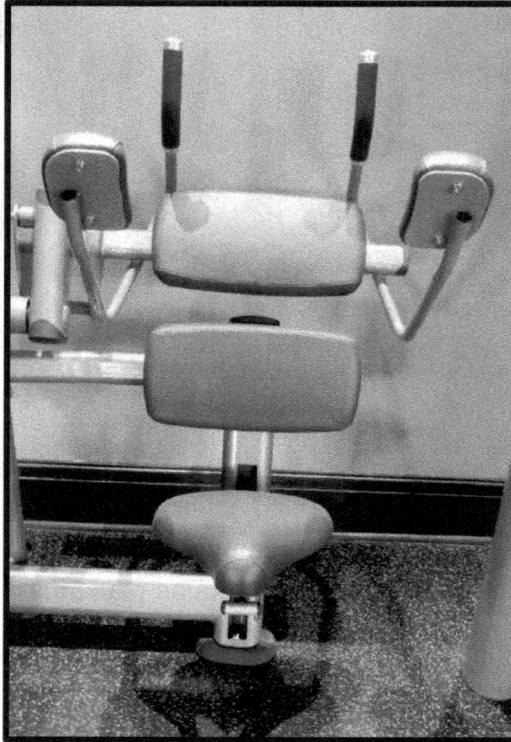

The Life Fitness Abdominal Machine, an
example of machines that work well with
Pain Free Functional Strength

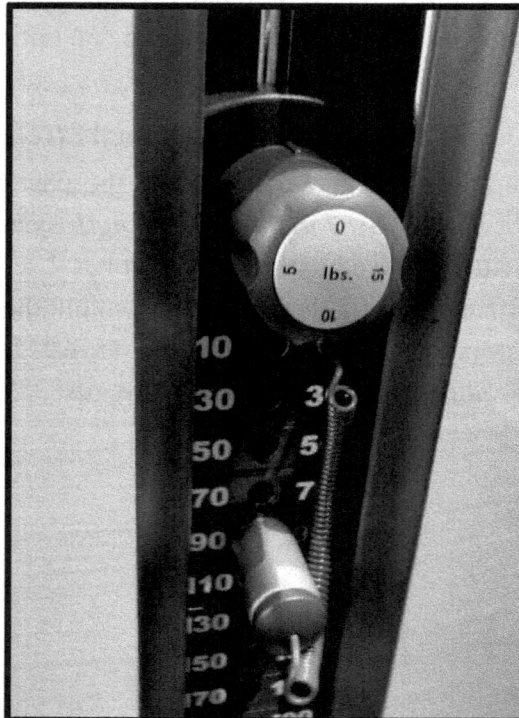

This machine has a dial on the weight stack
allowing for 5-pound increases – perfect
when on Pain Free Functional Strength.

Machines That Don't Have an Adjustment Dial:

If the machine doesn't have these more modern adjustment knobs, they may have add-on weights. These allow the exerciser to increase by a half of a plate instead of increasing by a whole plate. (See photos)

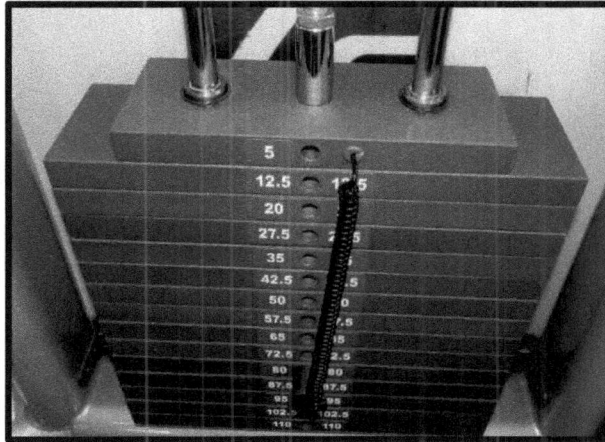

This is the top of a typical weight stack on an exercise machine.

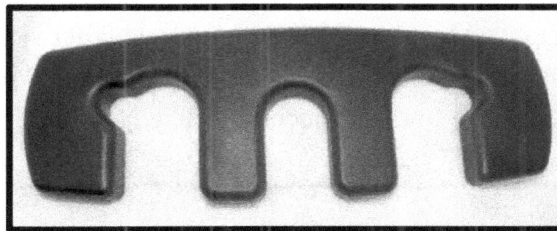

Here is an add on weight that is half the weight of the large plates

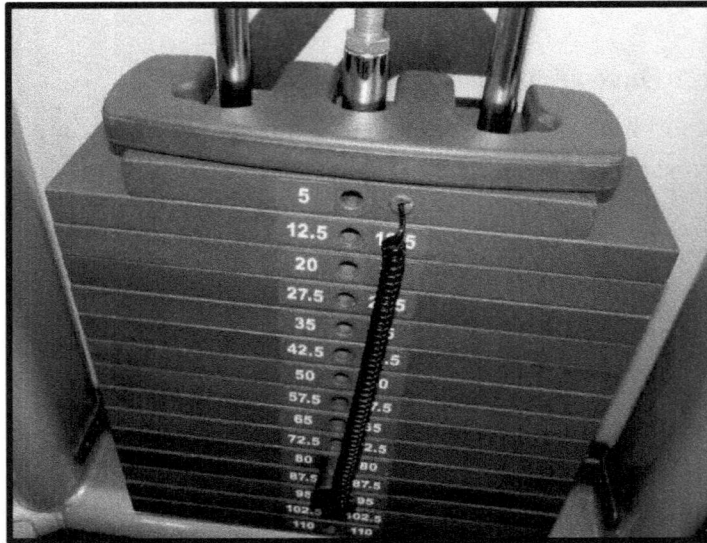

Here the add-on weight is placed on top of
the weight stack for a smaller increase than
adding a whole plate.

Plate Loading Machines

Another great choice for using machines for *Pain Free Functional Strength* is a line of machines called "plate loading" machines. This simply means that the exerciser can use weight plates from the gym for the desired weight. Most gyms have plates in smaller sizes such as 2 ½ pound, 5 pound and 10-pound plates. This makes them a great choice when on *Pain Free Functional Strength.* Below is a photo of a typical plate loading machine – The Hammer Strength Leg Press machine.

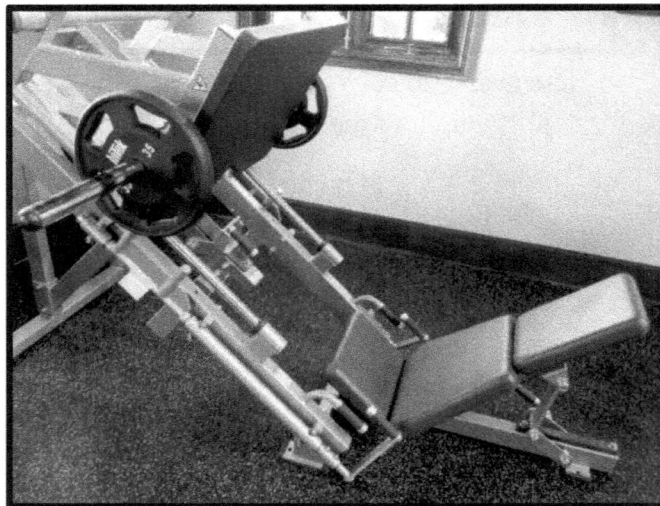

This is the Hammer Strength leg press.
Machines like these works well when on
Pain Free Functional Strength

Assisted Chin Up, Dip Machine

For the past 15 years or so these machines have been appearing in gyms across the country and they work well with the *Pain Free Functional Strength* system. Also, they are fabulous natural body exercises that have a history of getting great results. The problem with the traditional chin ups and dips is that they are way too difficult for most people. Because these exercises use your body weight for the resistance, the weight can't be changed like when using other exercises. That is until the invention of these clever machines – the assisted chin up and dip machine (either found separately, or together in one machine). These work well with *Pain Free Functional Strength* but one important word of caution – instead of adding or subtracting weight in the usual manner, it is exactly the opposite for most of these machines. When you add weight, the exercise gets easier when you subtract weight it makes it harder. Feel free to use these machines as an effective part to your *Pain Free Functional Strength* workout but remember to move the pin in the correct position to make the needed increase in difficulty.

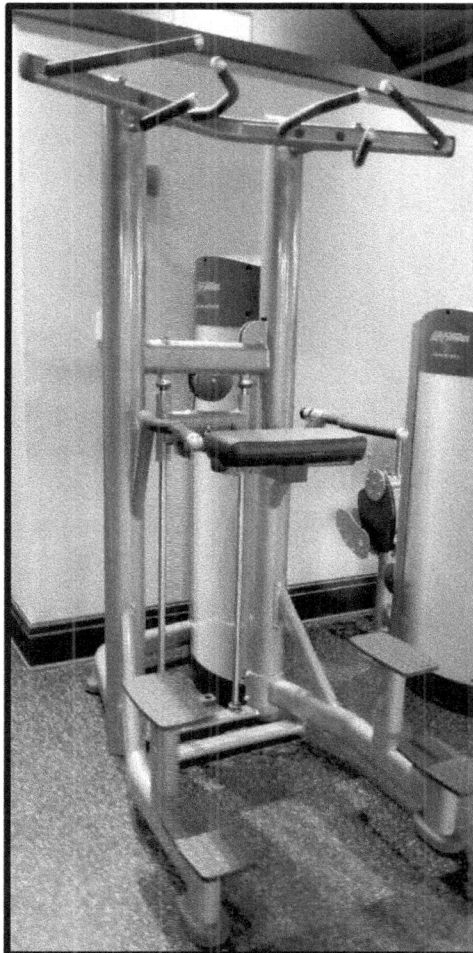

This is the Life Fitness Assisted
Chin up dip machine, another
exercise that works well when
on Pain Free Functional
Strength

Increasing Your Weights When Using 50 or More Pounds

In the above scenarios, we looked at many options to make the necessary small weight increases when using less than 50 pounds. Next, we will look at making increases when the weights are heavier than 50 pounds. This is much simpler because there is no need to find other options – you will be able to make the increases with weights the gym already has.

Here's a scenario where the user is working out with weights heavier than 50 pounds on the Hammer Strength bench press machine, but he or she wants small weight increases. (See photos) After 50 pounds, then the simple addition of the 2 ½ -pound, 5-pound, and 10-pound plates can be used. Just remember the goal is to try to increase in small 5 to 10 percent increments. This is one of the secrets of success in the *Pain Free Functional Strength* system.

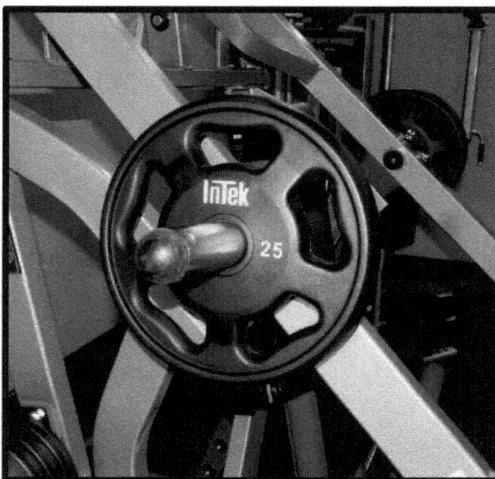

This user has just done 3 sets of
12 reps with 25 pounds on each
side of the bar.

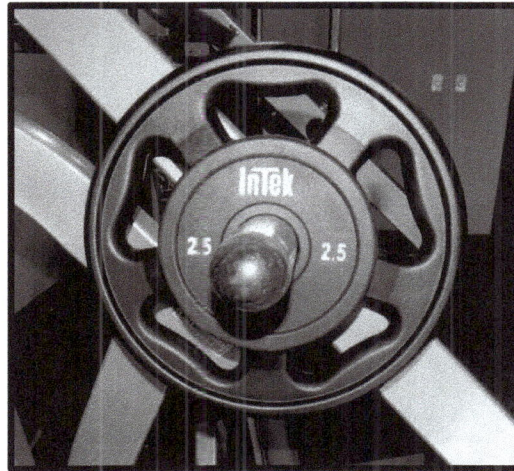

The user now adds 2.5 pounds
for the next workout, and does 3
sets of 8 reps

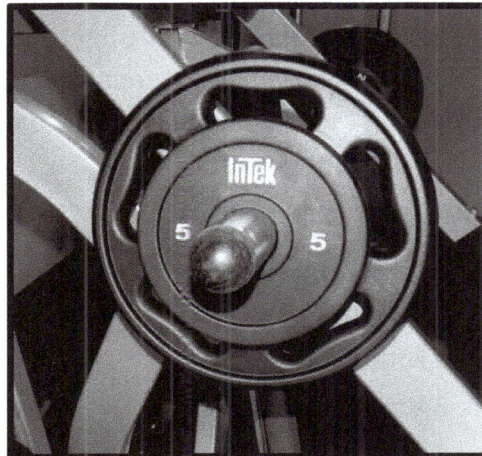

For the next increase the user
takes the 2 ½ pound plates off
and puts the 5-pound plates on.

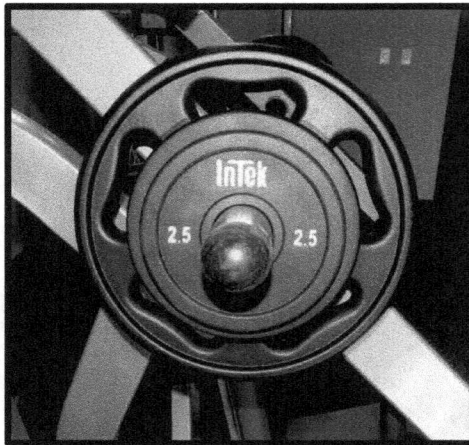

For the next increase the user
adds an additional 2 ½ pound
plate to each side.

This time let's look at another scenario that shows how the weights increase when on the **Pain Free Functional Strength** program when the lifter is using at least 50 pounds. Let's assume we have a male in his mid-twenties who has been working out for a few years. He is starting out on the bench press using a 45-pound plate on each side of the bar (the bar by itself weighs 45 pounds). His progression might look like this:

* Workout 1 – larger bar with a 45-pound plate each side. 3 sets of 8 reps

* Workout 2 – same weight, 3 sets of 9 reps

* Workout 3 – same weight, 3 sets of 10 reps

* Workout 4 – same weight, 3 sets of 11 reps

* Workout 5 – same weight, 3 sets of 12 reps

* Workout 6 – add 2 ½ pounds each side of bar, do 3 sets of 8 reps

* Workout 7 – same weight, 3 sets of 9 reps

* Keep going as long as you can using this method for increase.

Do you know how to do the math to know the percentage increase?

This would be easy if the amount of weight were 100 pounds even. A 5 percent increase would simply be 5 pounds. But what about scenarios where the weight is more complicated, like 35 pounds or 225 pounds? To figure out the percentage of an increase, you need to multiply the weight you are currently doing by either point 05 for a 5 percent increase or point 1 for a 10 percent increase. So, in the case of the first example of 35 pounds, a 5 percent increase would mean multiplying 35 x .05, or a 1.75-pound increase. A 10 percent increase would be 35 x .1 which equals 3.5 pounds. So, this exerciser, after successfully completing 3 sets of 12 reps, could make an increase of any weight between 1 ¾'s pound and 3.5 pounds.

Let's look at the other example, an exerciser wants to increase after he or she has successfully completed 3 sets of 12 reps at 225 pounds. 225 x .05 = 11 ¼ pounds. 225 x .1 = 22.5 pounds. This exerciser could increase, as closely as possible, from 11 ¼ pounds to 22 ½ pounds.

Whatever It Takes for Making the Proper Weight Increase - Conclusion

Whether you use dumbbells with the magnetic add-on weights or wrist weights, or the bar with one pound collars, Ader micro load plates, or the Plate Mates 1 ¼ pound plates, or the exercise machines, it doesn't really matter. Maybe you can get creative and come up with another option that I never thought of. Perhaps there are other products out there that do this that I haven't yet discovered.

2. How to Choose Exercises

Just about any exercise can be adapted to work with the *Pain Free Functional Strength* system. However, certain exercises do work better than others. For example, the bench press and bicep curls work great on *Pain Free Functional Strength*. On the other hand, trying to incorporate chin ups or dips into the workout is much trickier.

Keep it Balanced

If you're just starting out, I recommend you simply follow the workout for beginners found later in this manual. But for those of you who have some experience, you can set up your own routine or use the workouts I've included later on. If you do set up your own workout and want to use the *Pain Free Functional Strength* system, that's fine. Be sure you pick exercises to work your whole body. For example, don't do the bench press for your chest but ignore the exercises that work your upper back. Likewise, you wouldn't want to work your bicep muscles without also working out your triceps. The more you can keep your exercises in balance in this manner, the better off your muscular system will be.

Dumbbells, Bars or Machines?

The good news is that any one of these can work great with *Pain Free Functional Strength*. I've used all of these countless times with remarkable success.

Your Muscles Don't Care!

Those who work out will often get hung up on what type of equipment they should use to get the best results. The answer – they're all good! Your muscles don't know the difference between a cable bicep curl, a bar bicep curl, or a machine bicep curl. Your bicep only knows one thing – contract! Therefore, it doesn't matter what type of equipment you end up using.

Pick Exercises That Will Work

Since we've already established you can get good results using just about anything, you may need to look at other factors in making you final decision. For example, if you decide to use the machine bench press, will it allow you to make the small increases needed for *Pain Free Functional Strength* or does it only increase by 10-pound plates? Or you like the wide grip pull down for your upper back but have noticed that your gym only had one and it's almost impossible to get to it when the gym is busy. Consider all these factors before making your final decision on the exercises you choose for *Pain Free Functional Strength.*

From here we will move on to the actual working out portion of this book. The next chapter is crucial for getting your Pain Free Functional Strength program right; please read it carefully.

Chapter 6 – It's Time to Start the Workout, You Must Get This Right!

Setting Your Starting Weights

It's very important to set your starting weights at the proper amount. But how does one know how to do this? Not to worry, after reading this section you should have a good idea of how to correctly set your starting weights.

3 Choices for Setting Your Starting Weights

Because of differing personality types, I have discovered that people catch on to something quicker if it fits their particular liking. Some people are good with numbers, others dislike numbers but gravitate towards words or phrases. That's why there are 3 choices to get you started. One is not superior to the other, they are all equally effective. Just pick the one you like.

But whether you choose 1, 2, or 3, you will need to experiment on each exercise going heavier or lighter to find that ideal starting weight. Once you find it, write it down above the first spot in the *Pain Free Functional Strength* workout chart above the word "weight" for each exercise. That will be your official starting weight for that particular exercise. You will need to proceed down the workout chart doing this for each exercise.

Choice Number 1 – The 1 – 10 System

To illustrate this, let's say I was working you out and I had you do one set of 10 reps on any given exercise; we'll use the overhead dumbbell military press for this scenario. As your trainer I would want to know how difficult it was for you to get all 10 reps; that's where the 1-10 scale comes in.

If the weight was so light you tell me you believe you could go on and on almost effortlessly, then we would assign that a # 1. On the opposite end of the scale, what if the exercise was so difficult, it took all your might to get that 10th rep (but you were still able to do it)? We would give that a rating of # 10. Now do you see how it works? If it felt about in the middle of these two extremes, we might give it a # 5.

Using choice # 1, start your *Pain Free Functional Strength* weights at a number 4 or 5. It should be fairly easy to get one set of ten reps. Next, write down that starting weight on your workout chart which you'll find later in this manual. Go down your list and do this for each exercise.

Choice Number 2 - The Phrase Method

If you're not a numbers kind of person, this might be the method for you. If I had you do 1 set of 10 reps on any given exercise and I wanted to know how difficult it was I would have you pick one of these ten phrases that best matched how you felt.

- Way too easy
- Easy
- Fairly easy
- A little less than moderate
- moderate
- a little difficult
- pretty difficult
- very difficult
- extremely difficult
- nearly impossible, but you got it

Start your *Pain Free Functional Strength* weights at or a little less than moderate for each exercise. Go through all the exercises and find the weight that allows you to do 1 set of 10 reps on each exercise in that moderate range. Finally, write down these starting weights on your workout chart.

Choice Number 3 – Using a Maximum Lift (commonly called a "max")

Only experienced lifters should use this method – it is the hardest method of the 3 to find but it is the most accurate. A max is the most weight you can lift one time with no help. In other words, the weight is very heavy! I am not going to explain how to find the one rep max, rather I will leave this one to the experienced lifters. If you don't know what you're doing, this choice can be downright dangerous!

Using choice number 3, the one rep max, start your *Pain Free Functional Strength* program at about 45 to 50 percent of your one rep max. For example, if you did a one rep max of 200 pounds on the bench press, your starting weight would be 90 – 100 pounds (or 22 ½ to 27 ½ pounds on each side of the bar). Once you find these weights write them down for each exercise on the *Pain Free Functional Strength* exercise chart.

Also, if you decide to use this choice, don't think that you have to use it for every exercise. Some exercises don't work well for the one rep max like shoulder shrugs or calf raises. Others work very well like the bench press or the front pull down. Feel free to mix and match the other methods using the one rep max for just a few select exercises. *Pain Free Functional Strength* gives you this built in flexibility.

In Summary

Whichever of the 3 choices you decide to use, find the weight that is in the middle difficulty range for each exercise. Write it down on the *Pain Free Functional Strength* workout chart found later in this manual, and you are now ready for your first full workout.

Congratulations – You Are Now Ready for Your First Pain Free Functional Strength Workout

It's day one. You should have your *Pain Free Functional Strength* workout chart in hand ready to go, with the starting weights written in for leach exercise. If you're using weights less than 50 pounds on the curl bar, or the dumbbells, you should also be ready with one of the 3 options for making the necessary small increases in weight – the one pound collars, the wrist weights, or the Plate Mates.

Workout Number 1

In this workout you will do 3 sets of eight reps for each set at the weight you already wrote in. This first workout may have felt a little easier than you're used to; that's how the program was designed, and the lighter feeling is perfectly normal for *Pain Free Functional Strength.* Once you have completed the first workout, rest about 2 – 3 days before working out again. That will be the normal rest period when on *Pain Free Functional Strength* during the entire program.

Workout Number 2

Repeat what you did the last workout, but instead of doing 3 sets of 8 reps, you are now going to do 3 sets of 9 reps, at the same weights as the previous workout.

Workout Number 3

Same weights as the last workout but now do 3 sets of 10 reps.

Workout Number 4

Same weights as the last workout but now do 3 sets of 11 reps.

Workout Number 5

Do 3 sets of 12 at the same weight as the last workout

Workout Number 6

Things change now. Increase the weights only by about 5 to 10 percent on each exercise. Now do all your exercises at 3 sets of 8 reps.

Workout Number 7

Repeat what you did the last workout, but instead of doing 3 sets of 8 reps, you are now going to do 3 sets of 9 reps, at the same weights as the previous workout.

Workout Number 8

Same weights as the last workout but now do 3 sets of 10 reps.

Workout Number 9

Same weights as the last workout but now do 3 sets of 11 reps.

Workout Number 10

Do 3 sets of 12 at the same weight as the last workout

Workout Number 11 – Start of "even it out" weeks.

Raise the weights again by the same 5 to 10 percent. Back the reps down to 3 sets of 8 and do it all over again and again.

At this point in your *Pain Free Functional Strength* program, I strongly recommend taking this next step for the purpose of evening out your workouts. If you don't do this (and that's your choice, the program will work either way), then some of your workouts will all be 3 sets of 8 reps, 9 reps, 10 reps, 11 reps and most importantly, 12 reps. When the weights are on the light side, this is not as important. But when the weights get heavy this will become more and more important. When the weights are on the heavy side and you're doing all the 12 rep sets in the same workout, then naturally these workouts will not only be much harder than the other two workouts, but much longer as well.

Preventing this from happening is easy. Just use this following method, and to make it easier to understand, let's assume you're working out on Monday, Wednesday and Friday. On workout number 11 (Wednesday), you will be doing 3 sets of 8 for each exercise. But you're going to do something a little different than before. As you go through your routine, pick out about 1/3rd of the exercises that you would say are the most difficult of all of them. So, if you have 9 exercises, you would mark 3 of them that feel the hardest. Put some sort of mark like a letter H for "hard" by the name of the exercise. Continue with the workout doing 3 sets of 8 reps on all the exercises. When finished, you should have marked 3 of the exercises with an "H".

Workout Number 12 – Day 2 of "even it out" weeks

If you chose to even it out, continue your progression by doing 3 sets of 9 repetitions on each exercise for this workout (Friday), except those that you marked as the hardest the previous workout. Keep those three exercises at 3 sets of 8 reps, but do 9 reps on all the other exercises

Workout Number 13 –Day 3 of "even it out" weeks

Continue to do 3 sets of 8 reps on the exercises that you marked with an "H" two workouts ago. At this point there should be three exercises that you did 8 reps and 6 exercises that you did 9 reps on the last workout. Keep the exercises marked with an "H" at 8 reps, but progress to 10 reps for the other six. But like you did two workouts ago you will want to pay attention to how difficult the remaining six exercises are. Take three of those remaining six and mark by the name of the exercise a letter "M" for medium. At the end of this workout you should have done 8 reps for the three exercises marked with an "H" and 10 reps for the remaining 6 exercises. Three of the remaining six should have an "M" by the exercise name.

Workout Number 14 – Day 4 of "even it out weeks"

Continue to do 3 sets of 8 reps for the three exercises marked with an "H". Do 3 sets of 10 reps for the exercises marked with an "M". Do 3 sets of 11 reps for the remaining 3 exercises. For my personal workouts I like to mark these with an "E" for easiest.

Workout Number 15 – Day 5 of "even it out weeks"

This is the final workout for the process of evening out the workouts. Do 3 sets of 8 reps for the three exercises marked with "H". Do 3 sets of 10 reps for the exercises marked with an "M". For the remaining three exercises, perhaps marked with an "E", do 3 sets of 12 reps. At this point you have created a nice balance in the number of repetitions preventing the workouts being excessively difficult later on in the program.

Workout Number 16 and beyond

From this point forward the progression will remain the same. You progress go from 8 to 9 reps for the exercises marked with an "H", 10 to 11 reps for those exercises marked with an "M" and 3 sets of 8 reps for the reps marked with an "E", but a slight weight increase. Remember, each time you do 3 sets of 12 reps the next workout will call for a slight weight increase but back to 3 sets of 8 reps.

Do You Have It Now?

Hopefully you now see the pattern. Continue on this 8, through 12 rep pattern raising the weights for the next workout each time you successfully finish the 3 sets of 12 reps. Repeat the 8, 9,10, 11, and 12 rep pattern over and over again.

Here's How It All Ends

Continue on this pattern as long as you possibly can until the inevitable finally happens. The day will come when you find it impossible to get the number of reps that the workout chart called for. This usually happens on the 12 reps day. You get to try two times, meaning that if during one of your workouts you were not able to get your 3 sets of 12 reps, you get to try one more time during your next workout.

If you get the 3 sets of 12 reps, great job! You had to work hard for it. Now you can increase the weights and go back down to 3 sets of 8 reps for the next workout.

After You Reach the End – Now What?

So, you went through several cycles of 8 through 12 reps and finally reached the point where you could no longer get the number of reps the workout called for. Now what? For the following workouts, continue to get 3 sets of about 8 reps repeatedly from workout to work out on that particular exercise. You'll find that the exercises almost never all end at the same time. One or two will come to an end. The following week, one or two more, etc. So, while you're working the progression on the remaining exercises, keep doing those exercises that stalled out at any number of about 8 reps or more. But if you're feeling particularly strong in a workout, by all means go for the 3 sets of 12 reps even though you went 2 workouts in a row of not being able to get the reps that were called for. This rarely happens, but if it does, go ahead and make your weight increase and go back to 3 sets of 8 for the next workout.

Some other reasons you may want to end an exercise on *Pain Free Functional Strength*:

The normal way that an exercise ends is to not be able to get the prescribed number of reps for 2 workouts in a row. But there are 4 other reasons people sometimes wish to discontinue an exercise progression even though they are still able to get the reps. These are:

1. Getting too strong:

You simply don't wish to continue getting this strong on a particular exercise. The reason this is brought up is because there are a few exercises that seem to be almost endless in the level of strength you can obtain – a level you simply don't care to go to. Examples of these exercises are dead lifts; calf raises and shoulder shrugs. If you are finding that you have already obtained a high level of strength on these, or any other exercise, and you don't wish to get any stronger than stop the progression and continue to do a number similar to where you stopped, as you work the other exercises.

2. Form is getting bad:

You find your form is getting worse in order to be able to do the exercises. For example, while doing low cable rows you are continuing to progress as usual, but you are not able to pull the handles all the way to touching below the chest. Or on the bench press, you are now having to arch your back off the pad to be able to get the reps. These also could be signs that an exercise can come to an end.

3. Decide to discontinue and move onto something else:

Perhaps several exercises have reached their predictable end but there are still a few that haven't. At this point, some exercisers decide to switch all the exercises over to the 5, 6, and 7 rep cycle of the workout. Or you may decide to end the workout and switch to an entirely different workout system.

4. Aggravating and old injury:

Since working very hard during phase 3, maybe you are noticing an old injury starting to become irritated. It's fine to stop at this point and go on to something else.

After You've Reached the End of All the Exercises – An Advanced Technique

All of your exercises have finally come to an end and you're doing less than 3 sets of 12 reps on all of them. What now? At this stage you are probably seeing some great results and may not want to stop here. For you there is a way to continue.

Less Weight, Less Reps

That's right. To both confuse your muscles and give them a much needed break from the prior tough phase 3, you are now going to reduce the weights by going back 2 to 3 weight increases on the *Pain Free Functional Strength* workout chart you have been using. For example, if you maxed out at 150 pounds on the free weight squats, you would want to go back 2 or 3 weight increases – 135, 140, and 145 pounds. But now you will no longer be using the 8,9,10,11 and 12 rep scheme as before. You will change to a 5, 6, and 7 rep pattern instead. So now it looks like this: First workout- 5 reps at 135 pounds, next workout, 6 reps at 135 pounds, next workout, 7 reps at 135 pounds. The next workout you will increase by 5 pounds but go back to 5 reps. In other words, you are now on the same progression plan as when you did the 8,9,10,11 and 12 rep scheme as before. But as with the first round, it's a good idea to even out the workout to achieve a balance of 5, 6, and 7 reps in the same workout, as you did with the 8,9,10,11 and 12 rep workouts.

"But wait a minute – did you say decrease the weight and the reps?"

Yes, that's correct. In the usual way of doing things in the gym, this doesn't make sense. But when using the Pain Free Functional Strength method it makes perfect sense. By doing this, you will actually bring yourself from phase 3 to somewhere back to phase 1, but leaning towards phase 2. In other words, after you change from the 8 through 12 rep pattern to the new 5, 6, 7, once again your workouts will be much easier. This is not an accident – the program was designed to do this. Just follow the program and watch the great results continue. By dropping back the weights and reps you will be allowing the muscles and joints to catch back up from the strenuous phase 3 from before. But not to worry, the workouts will rapidly progress, and your body will be ready for the heavy weights that will soon be coming in the normal progression.

For Those of You That are Body Builders

You can do this one more time but be forewarned, you may put on more muscle than you bargained for! After you've gotten to the end of the second cycle of Pain Free Functional Strength and could no longer get your 3 sets of 7 reps, it's time to back it down once again – go back 2 or 3 weight increases from your previous workout chart from the 5, 6, 7 regimen and resume another cycle, but this time using 2, 3, and 4 reps. But use caution if you decide to go through this low rep cycle – the weights will be getting very heavy! Now it is strongly recommended that you do several lighter sets on each exercise before doing the 2, 3, or 4 reps that the program calls for.

But because you've worked for so long and hard the prior months, your body should be more than ready for these heavy weights. You've paid the price, now it's time to reap the rewards.

Chapter 7 – *After Pain Free Functional Strength, What Next?*

If you made it all the way to the end of a cycle of ***Pain Free Functional Strength*** and can no longer make any increases in weights or reps, congratulations! I know you worked hard, especially during the third phase when the going got tough.

You should be seeing some good results after all that effort. And you should be feeling much stronger now and have the increased confidence that goes with it.

The Best Strategy After Finishing the First Cycle of *Pain Free Functional Strength*

- Give yourself 4 to 7 days completely off from the gym. This will give your body some much needed extra recovery time.

- Start a whole new cycle of Pain Free Functional Strength using all new exercises.

- Put some variety in your workout using a different form of resistance. Did you do mostly machines? Try more free weights. Did you do all dumbbells? Next try a mix of machines and free weights.

- Try to go a little more advanced by using the technique described earlier – after the first round of Pain Free Functional Strength reduce the weights by 2 to 3 of your last previous progressions and start over again, but using 5,6, and 7 reps instead of 8,9,10,11, and 12 reps. Doing this will initiate the easier phase 1 all over again.

- Go back to another workout other than ***Pain Free Functional Strength*** if there was some other workout from your past that you liked. You can bring back ***Pain Free Functional Strength*** anytime now and make it a permanent part of your workout repertoire.

- Because there is such variety in machines, free weights, and dumbbells, and so many of hundreds of exercises, you could make ***Pain Free Functional Strength*** your only go to work out for your entire lifetime and still not cover them all.

Chapter 8 – Common Questions Regarding *Pain Free Functional Strength*

The following is a list of questions that frequently arise from people working out on *Pain Free Functional Strength*.

1. **How long should the rest period be in between sets?**

   The *Pain Free Functional Strength* system calls for 3 sets on any given exercise. The rest period in between sets should be no less than 30 seconds, up to about 2 minutes. But for those lifting very heavy, especially in phase 3, the rest can be much longer – even as much as 5 minutes. The key is, you want to be fully recovered before attempting your next set, but without having cooled off. This can be a tricky balance and is only figured out after much experience. In the lighter phase you may find that the 30 second rest is adequate, but as the weights get heavier more rest time is required.

2. **What about abdominal exercises – does *Pain Free Functional Strength* work for abs?**

   For some abdominal exercises yes, for others, no. Doing abdominal machines works well on *Pain Free Functional Strength,* but it's not a good choice for so many of the non-machine ab exercises like crunches, knee raises, and side crunches, for example. What I do with many of my clients is to have them do one ab machine exercise using the *Pain Free Functional Strength* system and then supplement with a variety of 3-6 additional ab exercises doing at least one set of 20-50 reps on each.

3. **It seems that using *Pain Free Functional Strength* is for just about everyone. Is there anyone it's not good for?**

   Yes, mainly those who are in a hurry to get results, and don't really care about taking more risks that come with this decision. Here's some examples: 1.) A model has a photo shoot in four weeks and needs to look her best in a hurry, 2.) A runner is competing in a road race in six weeks and wants to be peaking just before the race and 3.) Any boot camp situation like the military or fireman training where there is a very limited time for the purpose of getting the recruits in shape as fast as they can.

   Also, people who make a living out of being in gyms like fitness models and body builders would not want to use *Pain Free Functional Strength* as their mainstay, but it would be good even for these athletes as an occasional strategy for allowing the body to heal while still maintaining their strength or size.

4. How Long Does One Round of *Pain Free Functional Strength* Last?

If you set your weights correctly in the beginning, one typical round of *Pain Free Functional Strength* should last about 12 – 20 weeks. That is average but don't think you didn't get it right if it takes you a few weeks more or less. By the final weeks you should be seeing many of the exercises coming to their predictable end. If it goes shorter or longer that's OK as well. But the program can go much longer if you end up deciding to keep going with the 5, 6, and 7 rep counts, as well as the 2, 3, and 4 rep counts for taking it all the way. There is no official time frame to finish in – hey, if you're getting great results and enjoying the program there's no reason to stop.

5. Does one have to stay with the 8, 9,10, 11 and 12 rep count?

No. in fact there are a few exercises that I go a little higher on for the number of reps, mainly very short-range exercises and abdominal exercises. The four exercises I do this with the most are calf raises, shoulder shrugs, wrist curls, and the abdominal machine. Because on all of these the movements are only a few inches, I prefer to change the rep count from 8 through 12 to 13, 14 and 15. I normally do this on all abdominal exercises as well. You don't have to do this, but I think it's better to do more reps on these 4 exercises. To keep track of this adjustment on your *Pain Free Functional Strength* workout chart, just write 11,12,13,14, and 15 under the name of the exercise. So, when I cross off the 8,9,10,11 and 12 on the chart I know I actually did 11,12,13,14 and 15 reps.

6. Earlier in the book you mention a man who lost over a pound per day while on the *Pain Free Functional Strength* program. Is that typical?

No, I don't want to deceive anyone. If you just do *Pain Free Functional Strength* and don't also do a lot of cardiovascular exercise, and watch your diet, there's no way you're going to get results like these. For the man in that account, we did at least two hours daily of some form of aerobic exercise, mainly the bike, and I had him on a strict nutritional plan as well. The thing to keep in mind if you're trying to lose weight is that *Pain Free Functional Strength* is an excellent weightlifting program to be on while you're also doing cardiovascular exercise and closely monitoring your diet.

7. Isn't this workout too easy?

I hear this a lot, especially from those who have a lot of years with workout experience. *Pain Free Functional Strength* is very different than what most people have experienced. The workout is relatively easy the first few weeks, when compared to other programs. But this is one of the reasons *Pain Free Functional Strength* is so effective and safe. It allows the body time to change and adapt in line with the natural inner time clock that helps us to improve.

If you think the program is too easy after a few workouts, I urge you to stick with the plan and watch what happens. Use the easier phase to work on your form and allow your body time to heal. Before you know it, the weights will be getting harder. And then comes phase 3 and you'll be struggling with all your worth to get the numbers that the program calls for. Give *Pain Free Functional Strength* a full round before you quit – you'll be glad you did.

8. Is *Pain Free Functional Strength* considered a cardiovascular exercise?

No. It does give you some benefit, but it was not designed to be a cardiovascular workout. It is, however, strongly recommended that you do integrate additional cardiovascular exercise along with your *Pain Free Functional Strength* workout. How much? 20 minutes 3 times per week is a good start. But there's really no limit to the amount you can do. This number will be based on what your goals are. If you want to lose weight, the more cardiovascular exercise you are doing, the faster you will burn up the fat. That's of course, assuming that you are on a good nutritional plan as well.

9. How long should I rest after a workout?

As stated earlier, you will normally wait 2-3 days before doing your next workout. But if you are doing a split routine, where you work some of your muscles on one day and other muscles on another day, it is fine to work out several days in a row. For example, if you're doing a split routine you could work half your muscles on Monday and Thursday and the other half of your muscles on Tuesday and Friday. Wednesday, Saturday, and Sunday would be your rest days. On the other hand, if you're working all your muscles in one workout, your workout days could be Monday, Wednesday, and Friday, or Tuesday, Thursday, and Saturday. These are just examples. The most important thing is that you figure out what is going to work best for you and your schedule – then just get in there and do it!

10. Can I do more or less sets than the recommended 3 sets?

Yes. If your schedule doesn't allow enough time for the 3 full sets on each exercise, you can do 2 sets and still get good results. Just make sure you are covering all your muscle groups when putting together your workout – don't make the mistake of omitting certain muscles to shorten your workout time.

You can add sets if you want, but after 3 sets the law of diminishing returns kicks in, and you can't expect additional results in proportion to these extra sets. You would be better off adding more exercises, not sets, if you have more time.

11. I want to gain weight. Will *Pain Free Functional Strength* work for me?

It can, but I purposely didn't add this in Chapter 2 because if you want to gain weight while on *Pain Free Functional Strength* you must do some other things as well. This is a whole other topic, but briefly, if you want to gain weight on *Pain Free Functional Strength,* here are a few pointers. 1.) Do a minimal amount of cardiovascular exercise; 15 minutes 3 times per week would be plenty.

2.) Eat 50 to 100 percent of your body weight in grams of protein per day. For example, if you weigh 150 pounds you would want to be eating 75 to 150 grams of protein per day. 3.) Be sure you're getting lots of sleep. Take naps if you need also. 4.) Drink at least 8 cups of water per day and up to a gallon per day. 5.) Be sure to continue *Pain Free Functional Strength* past the 8 through 12 rep phase and go into the 5, 6, and 7 rep phase. From there you may want to go further and do the 2, 3, and 4 rep phase of the program. Do these things and it may surprise you how much muscle you can pack on.

12. Won't I lose my strength gains by dropping back the weights?

When you finish a round of *Pain Free Functional Strength* and want to start another round with different exercises, you will be dropping you weights back significantly lower. Likewise, this also happens when you drop back from 8 through 12 reps to 5, 6, and 7 reps, and then again to 2, 3, and 4 reps. I have discovered that with most people, not only don't you lose strength gains, but you surpass the place you would have been in if you just kept working out heavy. There's something about cycling heavy weight periods with lighter periods that seems to be superior to just lifting heavy all the time. The reason that this is so effective is that your muscles, tendons and joints get a much-needed break during the lighter phases. I urge you to give this a try. It may just shock you how much better results you obtain for the same amount of time spent in the gym.

13. Is it OK to drink water during my work out?

It's not only OK, it's required! Water drinking is critically important always, but especially during workouts. Muscles are about 70 percent water and it needs to be replenished often. Drinking about 2 – 4 cups of water during your workout will be beneficial to getting great results.

As far as sport's drinks go, save your money and stick to drinking water. It's the beverage of choice for getting the most out of your workout. And be sure to be drinking at least 8 cups per day. This is especially important when you are going through a round of *Pain Free Functional Strength*. Stay hydrated for best results!

14. How sore will I get when doing *Pain Free Functional Strength?*

This is one of the great features of this workout system. Because it starts out light and gradually builds you up, post workout soreness is not nearly as prevalent as with other programs. But I have clients report that they were a little sore initially, even though the weights felt easy. If a person gets sore from the light phase, imagine how horrible it would have been had they started heavy, like most programs have you do. As the weeks pass, you should have little to no soreness for most of the program.

Here's a great trick to use if you do experience muscle soreness after a workout. Take an Epsom's salt bath. Fill the tub with warm water and two cups of Epsom's salt. Relax in the tub for 15 – 20 minutes. Keep adding more hot water every couple minutes but don't make it uncomfortable. This age-old remedy works great for relieving sore muscles.

15. How do I resume if I had to take a break during Pain Free Functional Strength?

This was dealt with earlier, but briefly, *Pain Free Functional Strength* was designed in a way where it's easy to come back after an extended break. When life gets in the way and you have to take a week or two off, not to worry. Simply drop the weights back with 3 sets of 8 reps. But if you felt good and were in the earlier phase of the program, feel free to resume right where you left off.

On the other hand, if you had to miss an extended period of time such as a month, it might be better to start back at the beginning.

16. Is there a time of day that's more favorable for *Pain Free Functional Strength?*

No, this is completely dependent on what works best for you. If you are the type of person who is very busy, you may want to consider getting it done first thing in the morning. Doing your priority first is always best to ensure it actually gets done. But for some, they feel they get a better workout later in the day. As far as the body is concerned it just doesn't matter; just be sure you get it done.

17. Do I need to stretch or warm up before doing my *Pain Free Functional Strength* workout?

First, stretching. Stretching ahead of time is always a good idea before any strenuous activity, and it's almost a must before quick start-stop activities like tennis or racket ball. But from a practical standpoint, it's not totally necessary for *Pain Free Functional Strength.* If you have plenty of time, then it may be a good idea.

As for warming up, some people like to do 10 to 15 minutes, easy to moderate, on some form of cardiovascular exercise before starting their *Pain Free Functional Strength* workout. Next let's talk briefly about warming up for each exercise, more specifically. During the heavier phases such as phase 2 and 3, you might need to warm up for that particular exercise by doing a lighter set before doing the 3 sets required for *Pain Free Functional Strength.* For example, if you're supposed to do 70 pounds on each side of the bar for 3 sets of 10, it would be a good idea to first do a lighter set of 10 reps with just 35 pounds on each side. Do this for each exercise, if you feel the need, once the weights have reached this heavy stage.

18. Should I do my cardiovascular exercise before *Pain Free Functional Strength,* or after?

If you are combining your *Pain Free Functional Strength* workout with your cardiovascular workout, which should go first, or does it matter? This is another one of those topics that comes down to personal preference.

However, I would not recommend an intense, difficult cardiovascular session before your *Pain Free Functional Strength* workout, especially during the heavier phase 2 and 3 when the workouts are harder. Rather, you want your muscles to be fresh and strong so they can give you top performance during your *Pain Free Functional Strength* workout. But if you're going to keep your cardiovascular exercise on the lighter side, than it's fine to do it first. Let's not get too caught up in the details though. If you're doing both your cardiovascular workout and your *Pain Free Functional Strength* workout all at the same time – good for you! This shows how serious you are in spending the time needed to get yourself in great shape.

19. How fast should I do each repetition when doing *Pain Free Functional Strength?*

This is important. You never want to lift quickly, in a herky-jerky manner. Lift the weight smoothly and under your full control. Lower the weight back down a little more slowly than you lifted it. Be sure to go all the way up, and all the way down until fully extended.

Here's a little technique you can use to take your good results even a little further. Put a brief pause, about ½ second, at the top and bottom of each rep. When you do this, it forces the muscle to work a little harder by having to further control the movement.

20. Should I be breathing a certain way when doing my repetitions?

Breathing is also an important consideration. If you have high blood pressure, then you want to make sure that you don't hold your breath while lifting weights. If high blood pressure is not a factor, then that changes the rules for breathing during a workout. There is a natural breathing instinct within us that we all do, even though we were never taught how. It's called the Valsalva maneuver. Since this was born into all of us, it's a good thing to use when lifting. Simply stated, you breathe in quickly and then hold your breath during the hardest, heaviest portion of the lift, and then exhale when doing the easier, lowering portion of the lift. Why? Because when your lungs are fully inflated, they give more internal support to your muscles and spine.

Let's use the bench press, once again, for an example. You're on your back and have already lifted the bar off the rack so the bar is extended straight above you. The hardest part of the bench press is when the bar is next to your chest, up to a little past the half-way point, then towards the top it gets a little easier. This tough spot is often called the "sticking point" and a lot of exercises have one. So, to breath correctly on the bench press you would want to be sure your lungs were full of air on that hardest first half of the bottom of the lift, right past the sticking point. Therefore, you would breathe in as the bar was lowering towards your chest and have a chest full of air just before pushing up. Now hold your breath as you push up and beyond this sticking point. Once past the hard part, exhale, and then do it all again by inhaling as the weight once again approaches your chest.

Does this sound complicated? Don't worry. This is one of those things that if you think about it, you will probably mess it up. It comes very naturally; your body already knows how to do it instinctively and it comes in especially handy when lifting heavy.

21. Is it OK to mix exercises or do I have to do the 3 sets in a row?

It's preferred that you do your 3 sets in a row. But there are times when you may want to ignore this rule, for example, if the gym is crowded and you're in a hurry. In this situation, someone may have grabbed the 10-pound dumbbells that you were using, even though you only had one more set. It's perfectly fine to start another exercise while waiting for those 10-pound dumbbells in order to not waste time. Do what you have to in order to get through the whole workout in these crowded situations. Just remember, this is a workout for the rest of us; it's OK if things don't always go as planned.

22. Is a personal trainer needed to be on *Pain Free Functional Strength?*

Not as a rule because in a sense, you already have me as your personal trainer. In other words, when you decide to do *Pain Free Functional Strength* either alone, or with assistance, you have in your hands a well thought out, scientifically based, tried and proven workout where all the thinking has been done already. Now you just need to do it. Pick one of the six workouts in this book, follow the instructions carefully, and you're on your way to great results.

On the other hand, if you can afford the luxury of having a trainer, they can assist you in making sure you get through the plan as it is written. But if your trainer insists on pushing you and using the caveman approach, fire him or her and get someone who understands the wisdom behind *Pain Free Functional Strength.*

23. Should I check with my doctor before starting *Pain Free Functional Strength?*

Pain Free Functional Strength is one of the very safest programs out there – as close to fool proof as it gets. Even so, you may want to check in with your doctor before starting any fitness program, especially if you're over the age of 35. When your doctor sees the conservative nature of *Pain Free Functional Strength,* he or she will be thrilled to see a program that takes a person so carefully and methodically through the progression. Remember, it's your doctors that treat all the injuries as a result of the caveman approach.

24. Does the weight increase need to be the same throughout the whole Program?

No. Every time you successfully do 3 sets of 12 reps and you increase the weights, the increase does not need to be exactly the same. For example, you've been doing squats and you have been increasing by 5 pounds on each side of the bar for the first 4 increases. But now it's getting much harder and you want to slow down the progression. Feel free to start adding 2 ½ pounds on each side of the bar, instead of the 5-pound increases that you've been making. You can do this for any exercise at any time throughout *Pain Free Functional Strength.* Just be sure that you're not allowing the increase to go above the recommended 5 – 10 percent.

25. As a woman, I fear getting larger or "bulky" if I lift weights. If I do *Pain Free Functional Strength* is this something I need to worry about?

If you have that mindset as a female, you absolutely need to be assured that this program is not a women's "bulk you up" weightlifting program. In fact, if your goal as a woman were to get bulky, I wouldn't suggest *Pain Free Functional Strength.* This program is a great workout for toning the entire body, head to toe. Women who have done it see fat fade away and be replaced by a nice, well-toned, feminine physique. Work the program faithfully and do it as close to the instructions as you possibly can. Give it time and the results you desire will be soon to follow.

26. Do I need to stay within the 5 to 10 percent guideline for increasing the weight?

It is best to stay within the recommended 5 to 10 percent guideline, but there is some flexibility to this. As a general rule, it's always acceptable to increase by less than the 5 percent, especially when using very heavy weights. Reciprocally, it's never acceptable to make an increase of more than 10 percent. By doing that you would be abandoning the very crux of what makes the *Pain Free Functional Strength* workout so effective.

When using the micro-loading technique of using very small increases, it's not uncommon to increase the weight by as little as 1 or 2 percent. This is perfectly acceptable but is not written up in the program like this because doing this greatly increases the length of time a cycle of *Pain Free Functional Strength* will last. But if you're up for it, you can get amazing results if you don't mind taking the extra time.

In Conclusion

Everyone owes it to him or herself to complete one round of this tried and proven workout. For decades, I have seen it transform countless numbers of people ranging from the greatest super bowl champions, to the tiny housewife and mother of 3 kids. Stay within the guidelines as best you can – they have been slowly and carefully developed over many years and thousands of workouts. Don't let anything stop you from being the very best you can be. Keep in mind one of the most important rules, if something happens that temporarily sidetracks you, don't worry about it. Remember, *Pain Free Functional Strength* is a workout for the rest of us; it has been designed just for you. When the problems that life presents subside, get back in the gym without feeling guilty – you're doing your best. Stick with it and give each exercise your very best shot. How far can you go before finally reaching the end? You'll never know until you try.

Chapter 9 – Six Workouts Using *Pain Free Functional Strength*

The following are 6 different workouts that have been designed to use the *Pain Free Functional Strength* system. They are:

1. Beginner: Male
2. Beginner: Female
3. Intermediate: Male
4. Intermediate: Female
5. Advanced: Male (split routine)
6. Advanced: Female (split routine)

Pick a workout that most closely matches your experience level. But keep in mind that not any of these routines are harder than the others, it's just that the more advanced routines have more exercises, take longer, or have exercises that are more difficult to execute properly. The choices of exercises aren't what make *Pain Free Functional Strength* more difficult. The factor that makes the program harder or easier is how far you can take it before reaching the end (when you can't get the prescribed number of reps 2 workouts in a row).

Most of the exercises you will find listed are to be done using the methodology you have learned about in this manual. But you may find a few exercises that you will not do in this manner, rather, you will do them according to the additional instructions on the bottom of the quick sheet.

Each workout begins with a "quick sheet". Here you will find a quick recap of how to properly execute Pain Free Functional Strength.

The next page following the quick sheet will be the *Pain Free Functional Strength* workout chart. Use this to cross off the reps you do as you progress from workout to workout.

Beginner Male:

Pain Free Functional Strength Workout - Beginner Male: Quick Sheet – Review and Additional Instructions

Before Starting:

* Be sure you have a way to make small increases when using weights or dumbbells less than 50 pounds.

* Take one workout to get your starting weight established for each exercise. For all exercises, find the weight that you can get one set of 10 reps moderately easy.

* Write down all these starting weights on your *Pain Free Functional Strength* workout chart, just above the word "weight".

* Each exercise is explained in detail in the pages that follow your workout chart.

Pain Free Functional Strength – The Workout

* Your first workout – Do 3 sets of 8 reps for each exercise. (Except for the calf raises, abdominal exercises, shoulder shrugs and wrist curls. Instead of doing 8, 9, 10, 11 and 12 reps you will use 11, 12, 13, 14, and 15 reps for these exercises instead)

* Workout Number 2 – do 3 sets of 9 reps

* Workout Number 3 – do 3 sets of 10 reps

* Workout Number 4 – do 3 sets of 11 reps

* Workout Number 5 – do 3 sets of 12 reps

* Workout Number 6 – Increase the weight by only 5 to 10 percent for each exercise. But now drop your reps back to 3 sets of 8

* Workout Number 7 – do 3 sets of 9 reps

* Workout Number 8 – do 3 sets of 10 reps

* Workout Number 9 – do 3 sets of 11 reps

* Workout Number 10 – do 3 sets of 12 reps

* Workout Number 11 - Increase the weights by 5 to 10 percent once again on those exercises that you got 3 sets of 12 on during the last workout. Continue the normal progression on all the other exercises, or use the next 5 workouts to "even it out" (as described in chapter 6)

* Continue as long as you can using this pattern

* *Pain Free Functional Strength* ends on an exercise when you can no longer get the number of reps that the workout calls for 2 workouts in a row.

* For the remaining workouts, continue doing those exercises that came to an end for at least your 3 sets of 8 reps, while working the progression for the remaining exercises. When all the exercises

have come to their anticipated end, you have finished Pain Free Functional Strength –
Congratulations!

What now? Pick all new exercises and start back at the beginning. Or continue on this workout but decrease the weight by 1/3rd and do 5, 6, and 7 reps instead of 8,9,10,11 and 12.

Workout Chart – For 8, 9, 10, 11 and 12 reps Beginner – Male

(Cross off rep counts as you progress through workouts)

Exercise #1: Leg press Machine	Weight:	8,9,10,11,12		8,9,10,11,12		8,9,10,11,12
		8,9,10,11,12		8,9,10,11,12		8,9,10,11,12
		8,9,10,11,12		8,9,10,11,12		8,9,10,11,12
Exercise #2: Machine calf raise	Weight:	8,9,10,11,12		8,9,10,11,12		8,9,10,11,12
		8,9,10,11,12		8,9,10,11,12		8,9,10,11,12
		8,9,10,11,12		8,9,10,11,12		8,9,10,11,12
Exercise #3: Dumbbell Bench Press	Weight:	8,9,10,11,12		8,9,10,11,12		8,9,10,11,12
		8,9,10,11,12		8,9,10,11,12		8,9,10,11,12
		8,9,10,11,12		8,9,10,11,12		8,9,10,11,12
Exercise #4: Wide Grip Pull Downs	Weight:	8,9,10,11,12		8,9,10,11,12		8,9,10,11,12
		8,9,10,11,12		8,9,10,11,12		8,9,10,11,12
		8,9,10,11,12		8,9,10,11,12		8,9,10,11,12
Exercise #5: Dumbbell Military Press	Weight:	8,9,10,11,12		8,9,10,11,12		8,9,10,11,12
		8,9,10,11,12		8,9,10,11,12		8,9,10,11,12
		8,9,10,11,12		8,9,10,11,12		8,9,10,11,12
Exercise #6: Bar Curls, Regular Grip	Weight:	8,9,10,11,12		8,9,10,11,12		8,9,10,11,12
		8,9,10,11,12		8,9,10,11,12		8,9,10,11,12
		8,9,10,11,12		8,9,10,11,12		8,9,10,11,12
Exercise #7: Dumbbell Shrugs (10,11,12,13,14 reps)	Weight:	10,11,12,13,14		10,11,12,13,14		10,11,12,13,14
		10,11,12,13,14		10,11,12,13,14		10,11,12,13,14
		10,11,12,13,14		10,11,12,13,14		10,11,12,13,14
Exercise #8: Abdominal Machine (10,11,12,13,14 reps)	Weight:	8,9,10,11,12		8,9,10,11,12		8,9,10,11,12
		8,9,10,11,12		8,9,10,11,12		8,9,10,11,12
		8,9,10,11,12		8,9,10,11,12		8,9,10,11,12
Exercise #9: Low Back Machine	Weight:	8,9,10,11,12		8,9,10,11,12		8,9,10,11,12
		8,9,10,11,12		8,9,10,11,12		8,9,10,11,12
		8,9,10,11,12		8,9,10,11,12		8,9,10,11,12

Leg Press Machine

Target Area: Quadriceps (front of upper legs)

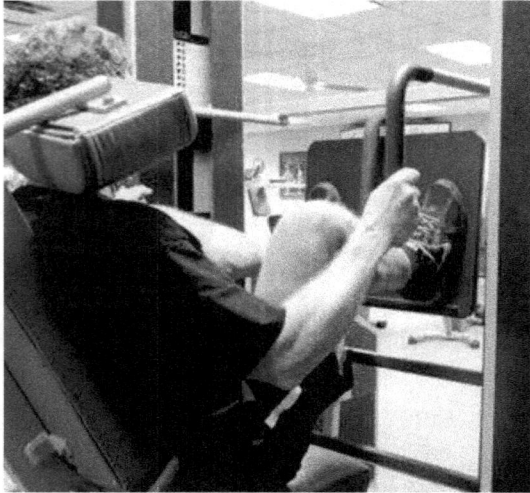

Start

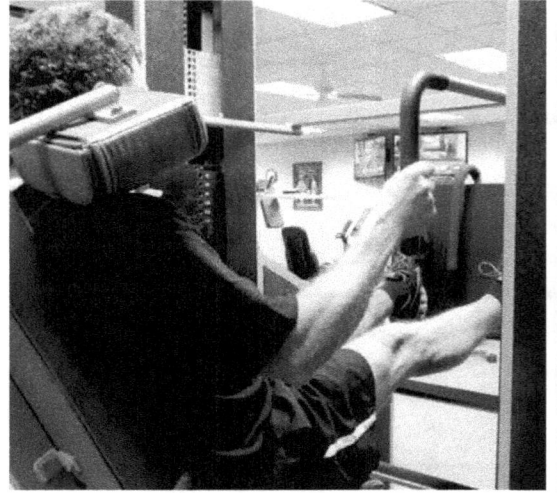

Finish

- Align the seat position so you can bring your legs back to about a 90-degree bend at the knees.
- Push with both legs equally until the foot pad is extended forward, but not so far as to lock your knees.
- Come back to start position and continue is this manner.

Mike's Special Pointer:

The leg press is an excellent machine, but the user must be very careful to keep the lower back well supported by ensuring that it is firmly pressed against the back seat.

Calf Raises - Leg Press Machine

TARGET AREA -   Calves - back of lower legs

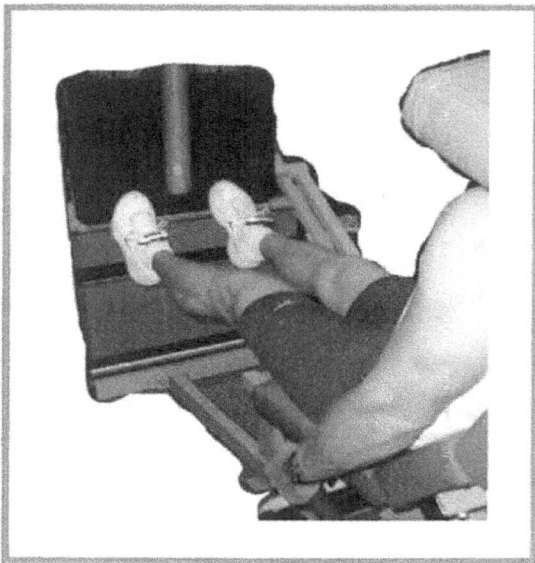

Start

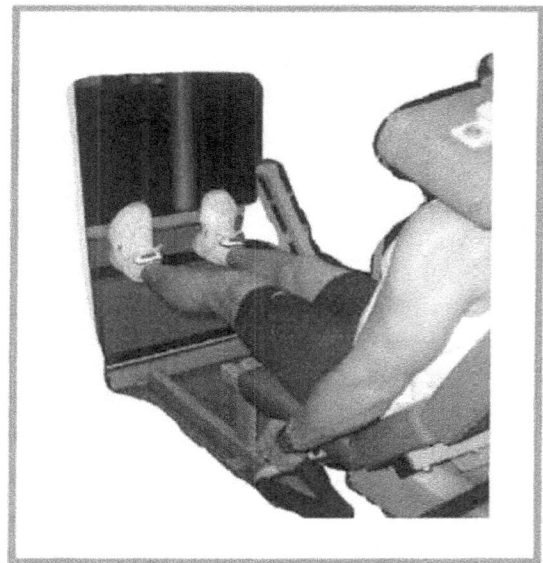

Finish

* Use a standard leg press machine, but be sure it is compatible for doing calf raises.
* Set the seat position so you can do a full range of motion on the calf raise without the weight touching back down after each repetition.
* Place your feet so that the upper 1/3 of your feet are on the foot pad.
* Push your toes forward as if you are trying to stand on your toes.
* Next, bring your toes back towards you until you feel a good stretch.
* Your knees should be only slightly bent the whole time.

Mike's Special Pointer:
You may need to readjust your feet every 3 or 4 repetitions - they tend to slide down as you do this exercise.

Dumbbell Bench Press

Target Area – Pectorals (chest)

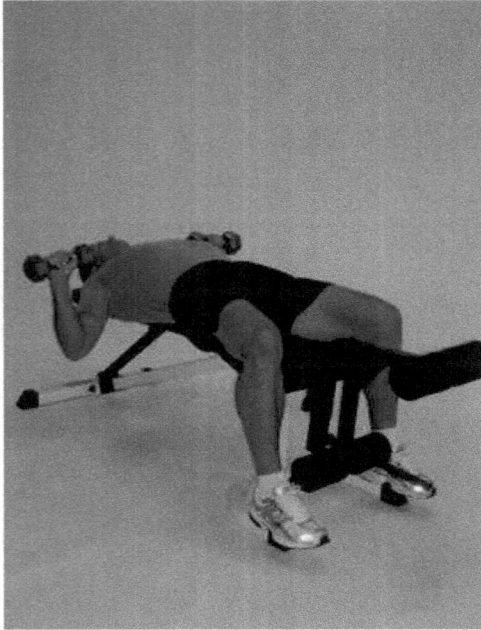

Start

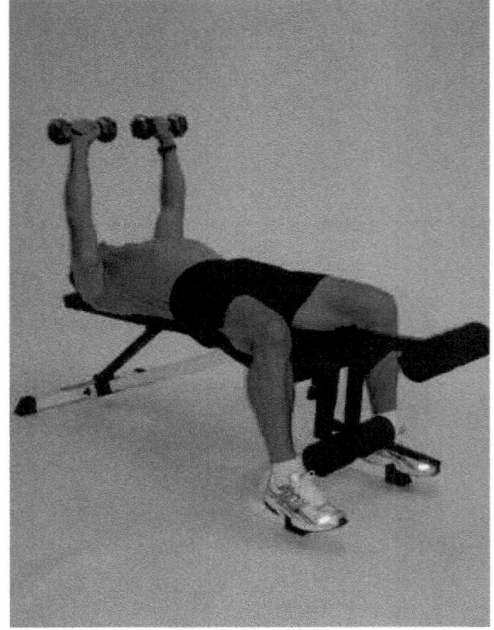

Finish

- Lay flat on your back, putting your feet up is optional.
- Start with the weights wider than your shoulders, elbows at or slightly below the bench.
- Push up and allow the weights to come close together at the top without touching.
- Don't lock out your elbows.
- Come back down to the start position, but don't let your forearms angle out – keep them straight up.

Mike's Special Pointer:

When pushing up, it's OK if your elbows are slightly forward. Many people can develop shoulder injuries if they try and force their elbows way back while doing the exercise.

Pull Downs: Front

Target Area – Latissimus (middle and outer back)

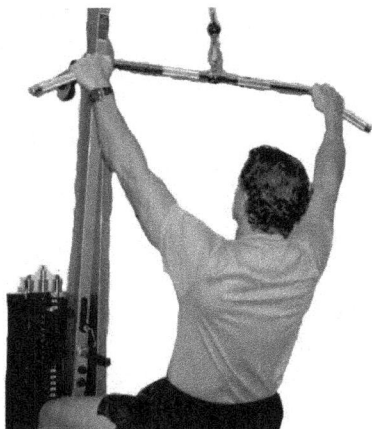

Start

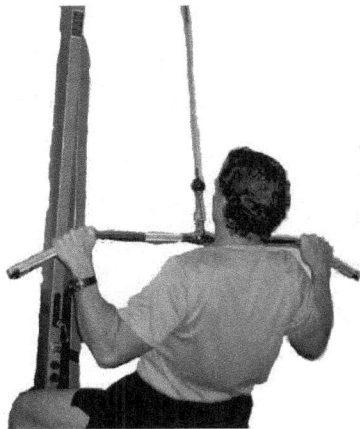

Finish

- Position hands wider than your shoulders, palms facing out forward, away from you.
- Pull straight down until the bar comes at or below your chin.
- Raise the bar back up to the starting position, be sure your arms are fully extended giving you a full stretch.

Mike's Special Pointer:

When coming down, don't turn your forearms down so that your palms angle down. When in the finish position, your palms should be facing straight ahead

Dumbbell Military Press: Seated

Target Area – Deltoids (shoulders)

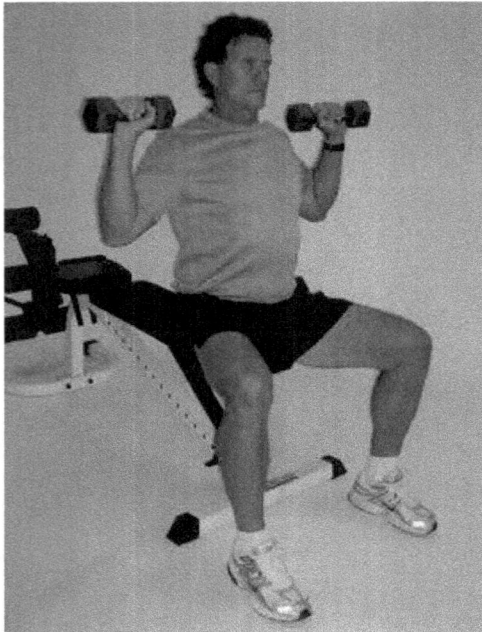

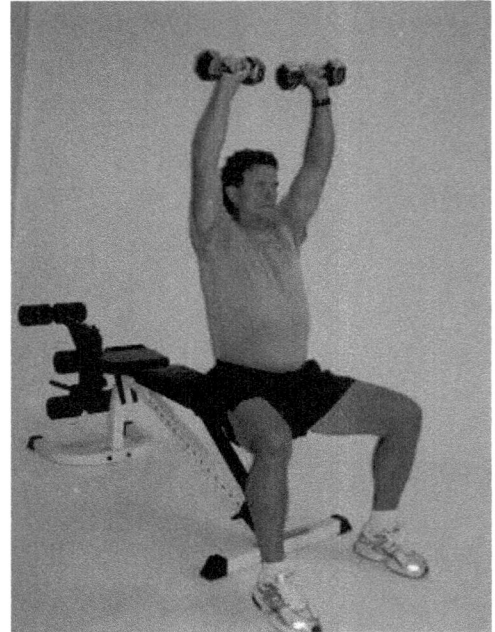

Start　　　　　　　　　　　　　**Finish**

- Hold the dumbbells just wider than your shoulders, with the weights parallel to the floor.
- Push the weights up, and the hands will naturally come closer to each other as you get higher and higher.
- Raise the weights until the elbows are just short of locking out.
- Lower the weights back down to the start position.

Mike's Special Pointer:

Make sure your back is supported by the back rest if the bench you are using has one. Keep your head and neck relaxed as you push the weight over your head.

Bicep Curls - Bar - Regular Grip

TARGET AREA -   Biceps - front of upper arms

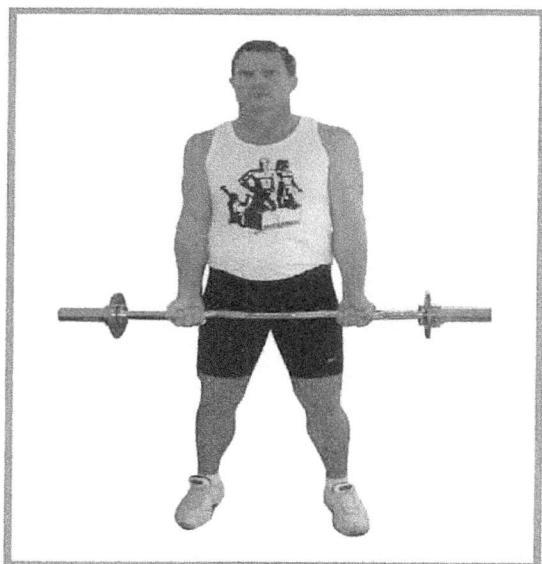

Start

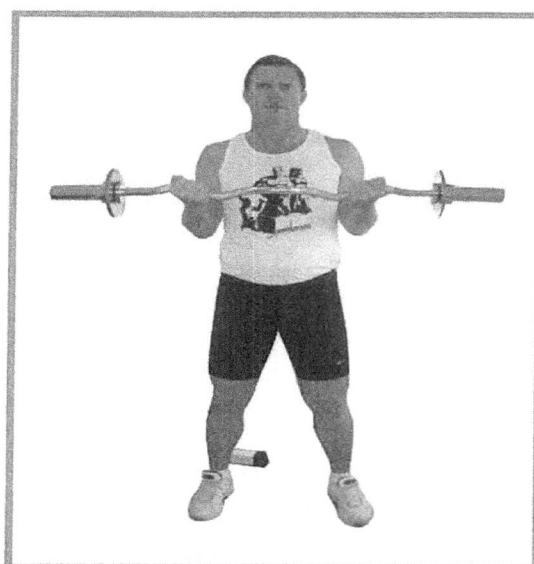

Finish

* Grab bar a little wider than shoulder width- special curl bar should allow palms to turn in slightly, feet about shoulder's width apart, soft knees.
* Keeping elbows down, curl the bar up towards the top of chest.
* Lower it back to start position.

Mike's Special Pointer:
Perhaps the most common mistake on bar curls is to bring the elbows forward at the top of the movement. This takes a lot of stress off the bicep muscle and puts it in the joint- exactly what you don't want when you do curls.

Dumbbell Shrugs

Target Area: Trapezius (upper back)

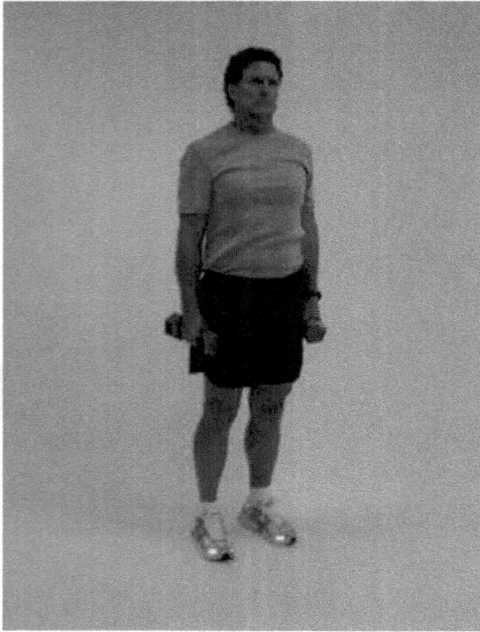

Start

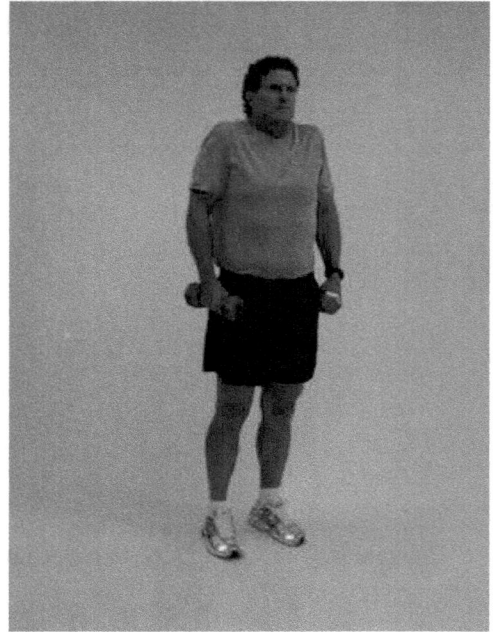

Finish

- Stand holding dumbbells at your sides, feet close together, knees slightly bent, palms facing in.
- Shrug your shoulders up as high as you can with hardly any bend of the elbows.
- Come back down to a full stretch at the bottom.

Mike's Special Pointer:

Dumbbell shrugs have one advantage over regular bar shrugs. You can move the weight forward or backwards a little until you feel it the best, whereas the bar only allows you one angle.

Abdominal Machine

TARGET AREA -   **Abdominals - front of torso**

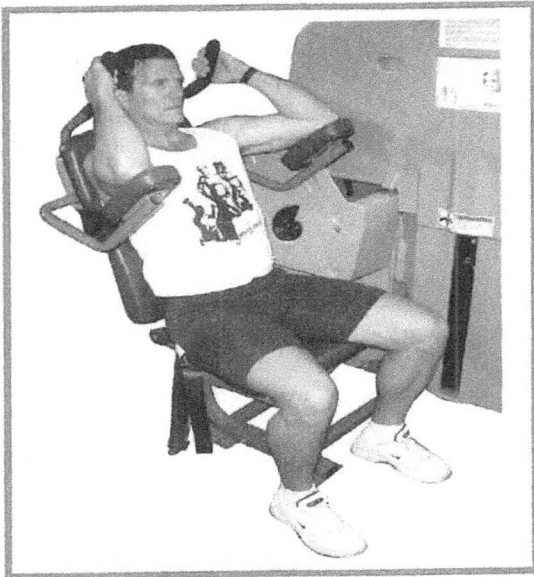

Start

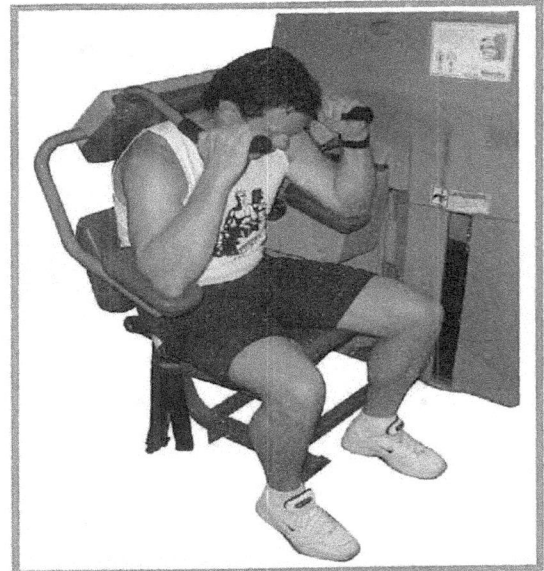

Finish

* Set seat so that your navel is about in line with axis of rotating arm of machine.
* Sit in seat, grab handles (if available), feet flat on floor, sit upright.
* Using your abdominal muscles, pull forward and then down.
* Return to starting position.

Mike's Special Pointer:
Don't allow your back to come out of the seat- keep it back at all times.

Lower Back Machine

TARGET AREA -   Lower Back

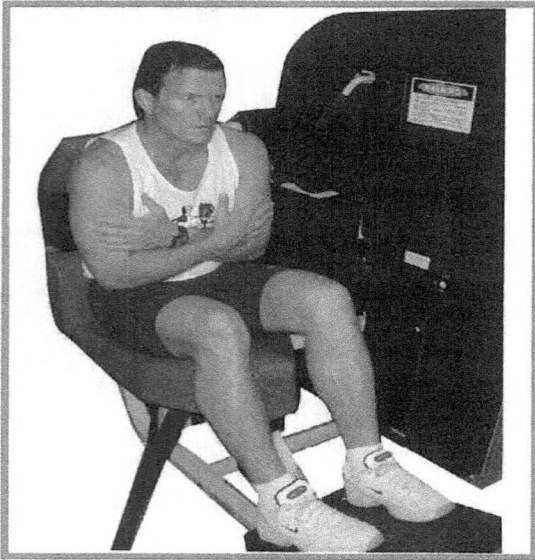

Start

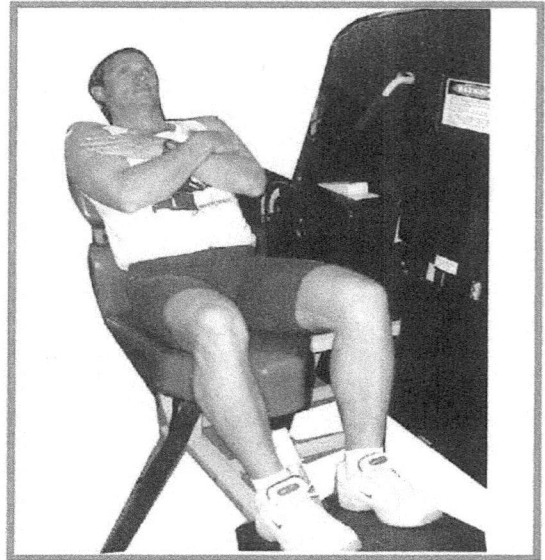

Finish

*   Set foot pad so knees are comfortably bent. Sit in machine, cross hands over chest.
*   Push back until legs and body are straight or until weight touches at top (depending on which style of machine you use).
*   Come forward to a stretch, or until weight touches back down.

Mike's Special Pointer:
Careful on this machine- it 's a good exercise, but don't try and lift heavy at first. Start light, and gradually progress as the weeks pass.

Beginner Female:

Pain Free Functional Strength Workout - Beginner Female: Quick Sheet – Review and Additional Instructions

Before Starting:

* Be sure you have a way to make small increases when using weights or dumbbells less than 50 pounds.

* Take one workout to get your starting weight established for each exercise. For all exercises, find the weight that you can get one set of 10 reps moderately easy.

* Write down all these starting weights on your *Pain Free Functional Strength* workout chart, just above the word "weight".

* Each exercise is explained in detail in the pages that follow your workout chart.

Pain Free Functional Strength – The Workout

* Your first workout – Do 3 sets of 8 reps for each exercise. (Except for the calf raises, abdominal exercises, shoulder shrugs and wrist curls. Instead of doing 8, 9, 10, 11 and 12 reps you will use 11, 12, 13, 14, and 15 reps for these exercises instead)

* Workout Number 2 – do 3 sets of 9 reps

* Workout Number 3 – do 3 sets of 10 reps

* Workout Number 4 – do 3 sets of 11 reps

* Workout Number 5 – do 3 sets of 12 reps

* Workout Number 6 – Increase the weight by only 5 to 10 percent for each exercise. But now drop your reps back to 3 sets of 8

* Workout Number 7 – do 3 sets of 9 reps

* Workout Number 8 – do 3 sets of 10 reps

* Workout Number 9 – do 3 sets of 11 reps

* Workout Number 10 – do 3 sets of 12 reps

* Workout Number 11 - Increase the weights by 5 to 10 percent once again on those exercises that you got 3 sets of 12 on during the last workout. Continue the normal progression on all the other exercises, or use the next 5 workouts to "even it out" (as described in chapter 6)

* Continue as long as you can using this pattern

* *Pain Free Functional Strength* ends on an exercise when you can no longer get the number of reps that the workout calls for 2 workouts in a row.

*   For the remaining workouts, continue doing those exercises that came to an end for at least your 3 sets of 8 reps, while working the progression for the remaining exercises. When all the exercises have come to their anticipated end, you have finished ***Pain Free Functional Strength*** – Congratulation

What now? Pick all new exercises and start back at the beginning. Or continue on this workout but decrease the weight by 1/3rd and do 5, 6, and 7 reps instead of 8 through 12.

Workout Chart – For 8, 9, 10, 11 and 12 reps Beginner – Female

(Cross off rep counts as you progress through workouts)

Exercise	Weight:		
Exercise #1: Leg press Machine	8,9,10,11,12 _____ 8,9,10,11,12 _____ 8,9,10,11,12	8,9,10,11,12 _____ 8,9,10,11,12 _____ 8,9,10,11,12	8,9,10,11,12 _____ 8,9,10,11,12 _____ 8,9,10,11,12
Exercise #2: Machine calf raise (10,11,12,13,14 reps)	10,11,12,13,14 _____ 10,11,12,13,14 _____ 10,11,12,13,14	10,11,12,13,14 _____ 10,11,12,13,14 _____ 10,11,12,13,14	10,11,12,13,14 _____ 10,11,12,13,14 _____ 10,11,12,13,14
Exercise #3: Bench Press Machine	8,9,10,11,12 _____ 8,9,10,11,12 _____ 8,9,10,11,12	8,9,10,11,12 _____ 8,9,10,11,12 _____ 8,9,10,11,12	8,9,10,11,12 _____ 8,9,10,11,12 _____ 8,9,10,11,12
Exercise #4: Machine Rows	8,9,10,11,12 _____ 8,9,10,11,12 _____ 8,9,10,11,12	8,9,10,11,12 _____ 8,9,10,11,12 _____ 8,9,10,11,12	8,9,10,11,12 _____ 8,9,10,11,12 _____ 8,9,10,11,12
Exercise #5: Machine Military Press	8,9,10,11,12 _____ 8,9,10,11,12 _____ 8,9,10,11,12	8,9,10,11,12 _____ 8,9,10,11,12 _____ 8,9,10,11,12	8,9,10,11,12 _____ 8,9,10,11,12 _____ 8,9,10,11,12
Exercise #6: Bar Bicep Curls	8,9,10,11,12 _____ 8,9,10,11,12 _____ 8,9,10,11,12	8,9,10,11,12 _____ 8,9,10,11,12 _____ 8,9,10,11,12	8,9,10,11,12 _____ 8,9,10,11,12 _____ 8,9,10,11,12
Exercise #8: Cable Triceps Extensions	8,9,10,11,12 _____ 8,9,10,11,12 _____ 8,9,10,11,12	8,9,10,11,12 _____ 8,9,10,11,12 _____ 8,9,10,11,12	8,9,10,11,12 _____ 8,9,10,11,12 _____ 8,9,10,11,12
Exercise #9: Abdominal Machine (10,11,12,13,14 reps)	10,11,12,13,14 _____ 10,11,12,13,14 _____ 10,11,12,13,14	10,11,12,13,14 _____ 10,11,12,13,14 _____ 10,11,12,13,14	10,11,12,13,14 _____ 10,11,12,13,14 _____ 10,11,12,13,14
Exercise #10: Lower Back Machine	8,9,10,11,12 _____ 8,9,10,11,12 _____ 8,9,10,11,12	8,9,10,11,12 _____ 8,9,10,11,12 _____ 8,9,10,11,12	8,9,10,11,12 _____ 8,9,10,11,12 _____ 8,9,10,11,12

Leg Press Machine

Target Area: Quadriceps (front of upper legs)

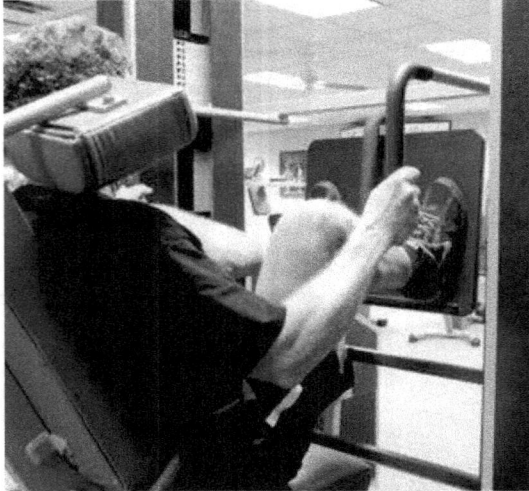

Start

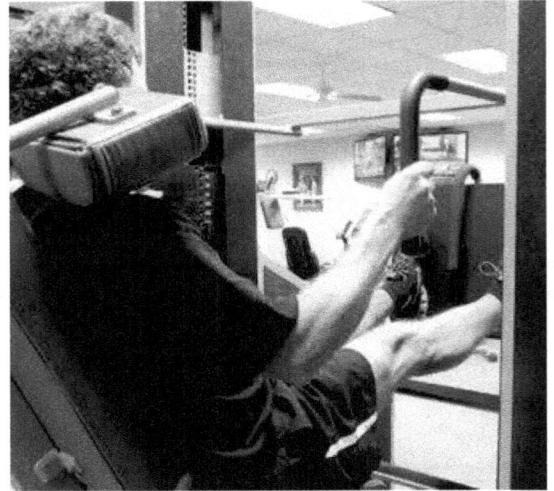

Finish

- Align the seat position so you can bring your legs back to about a 90 degree bend at the knees.
- Push with both legs equally until the foot pad is extended forward, but not so far as to lock your knees.
- Come back to start position and continue is this manner.

Mike's Special Pointer:

The leg press is an excellent machine, but the user must be very careful to keep the lower back well supported by ensuring that it is firmly pressed against the back seat.

Calf Raise Machine - Standing

TARGET AREA -   Calves - back of lower legs

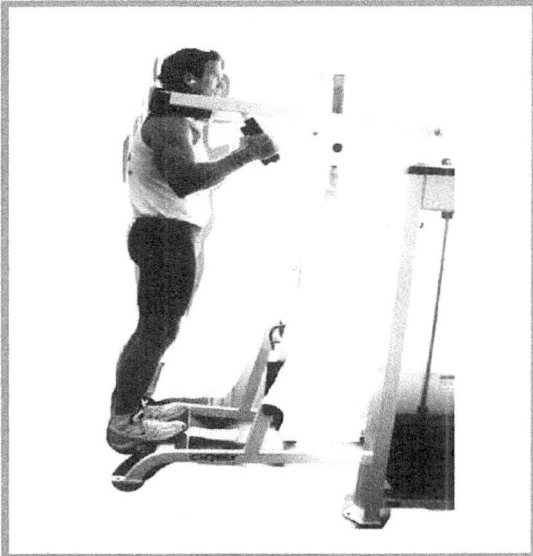
Start

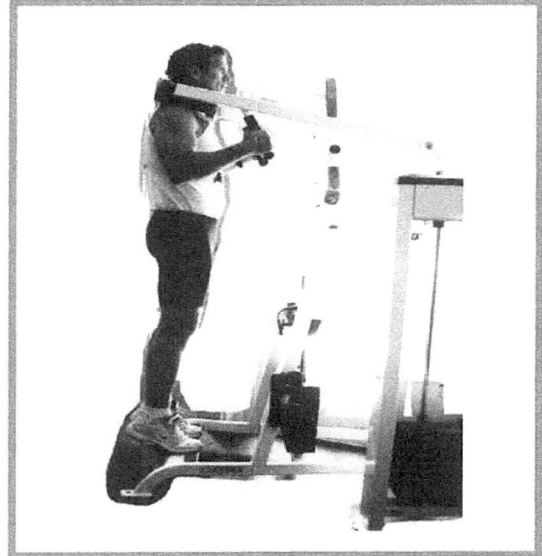
Finish

* Set machine so that you're able to go all the way up and all the way down without the weight stack touching the top or bottom.
* Get under shoulder pads, keep your back straight and lift the weight stack initially by pressing with your legs, not by bending your back.
* Position your feet so that the balls of your feet are on the step, heels hanging over, grab hand grips.
* Allow your calves to stretch fully by bringing your heels as close to the ground as possible, push up onto the balls of your feet as high as possible and pause briefly. Come back to a full stretch.

Mike's Special Pointer:
Keep a very slight bend in your knees while doing this exercise and keep it there for the entire time both up and down. Also, pause at top for at least ½ second for maximum effectiveness.

Bench Press Machine - Seated

TARGET AREA -   Pectorals - Chest

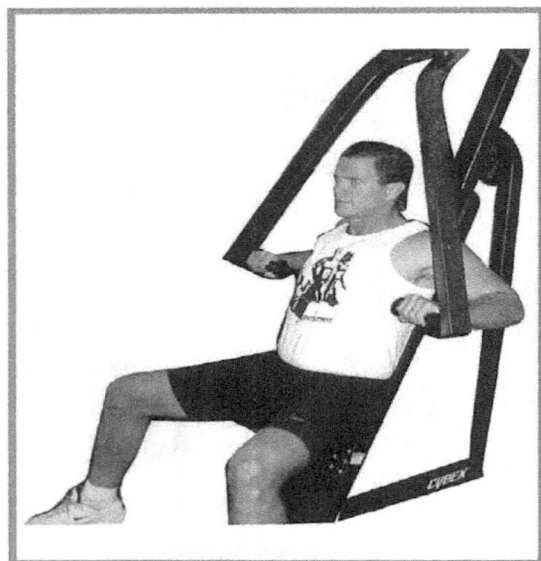

Start

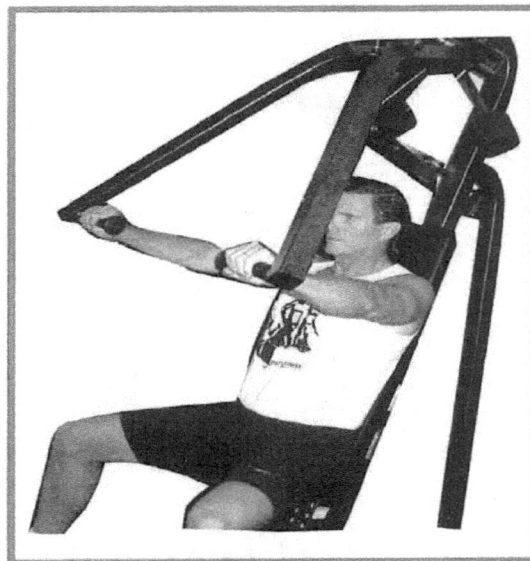

Finish

* Position seat so that when you grab the handle, they are at about the level of your lower chest, sit in seat, back firmly against pad.
* Start with arms extended but don't allow the elbows to lock, palms facing down.
* Come back to a full stretch, hands will be near chest.
* Push back to start position.

Mike's Special Pointer:
This is a good exercise to prepare for the free weight bench press if you're new to exercise. Also, opt for this if there's no one to spot you and you're lifting heavy.

Machine Rows

TARGET AREA -   Latisimus - middle and outer back

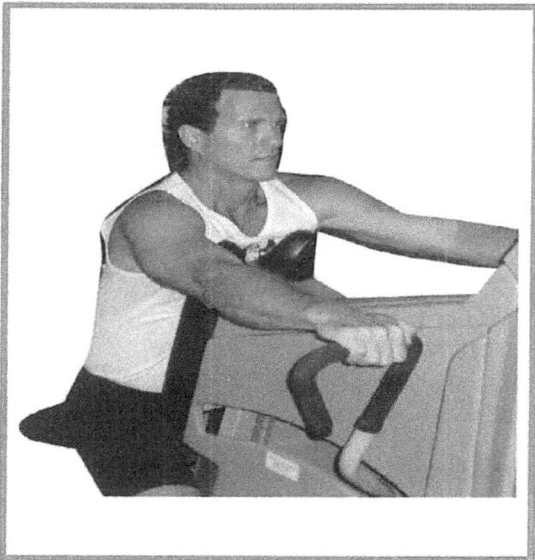

Start

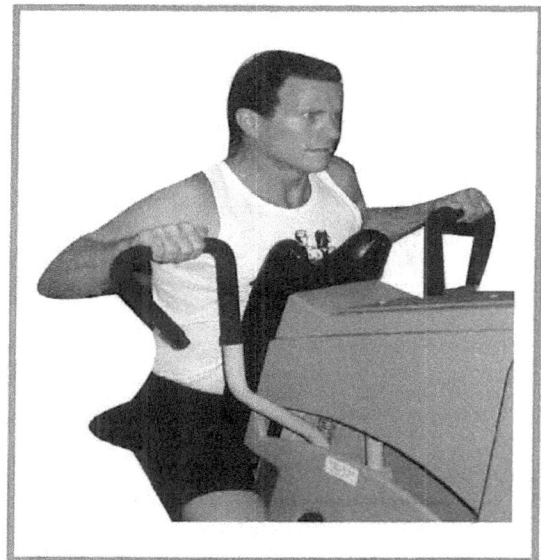

Finish

* Position seat so when you sit down handles will be at about chest level.
* Sit down facing the machine, grab handles with palms down,
  allow full stretch of your arms.
* Pull straight back, keeping your elbows up high.
* Return to start position.

Mike's Special Pointer:
Most Machines allow for different hand positions. Try different grips occasionally,
to hit your muscles a little differently.

Military Press - Machine

TARGET AREA -   **Deltoids - shoulders**

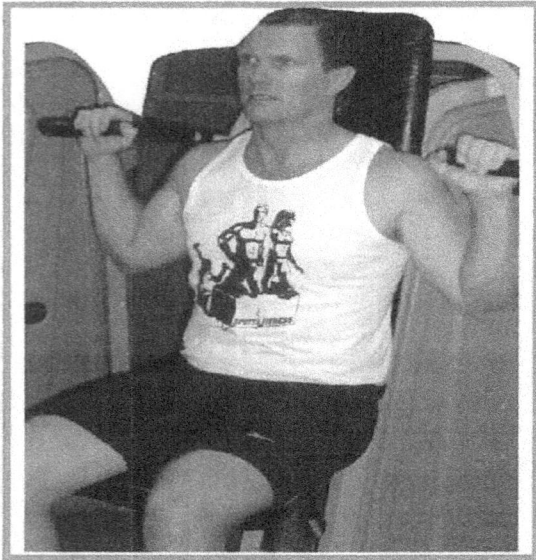

Start

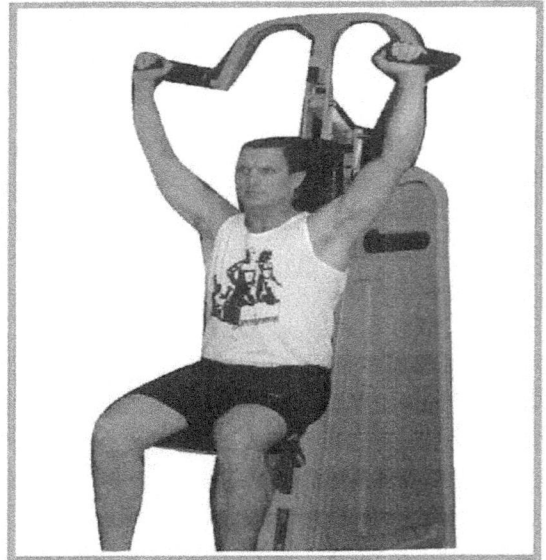

Finish

* Set seat so you can set and grab handles at about shoulder level, palms facing out.
* Push up until arms almost straighten.
* Come back to start position.

Mike's Special Pointer:
Never look to the side while doing this exercise, or any military press exercise - it can cause a neck strain. Find a relaxed position for your neck by moving your chin up and down to find just the right position for you.

Bicep Curls - Bar - Regular Grip

TARGET AREA -   Biceps - front of upper arms

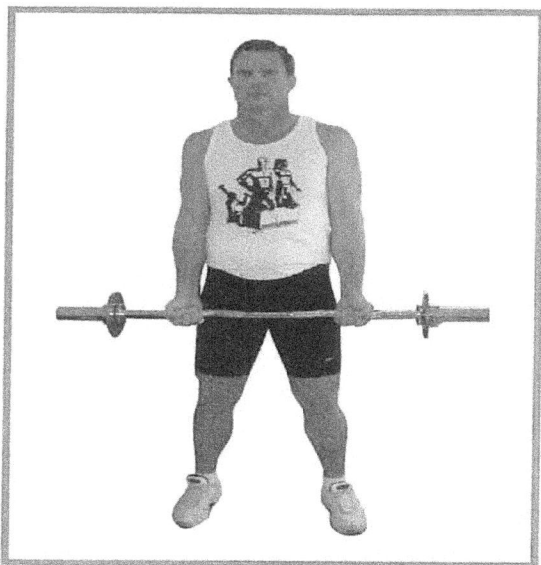

Start

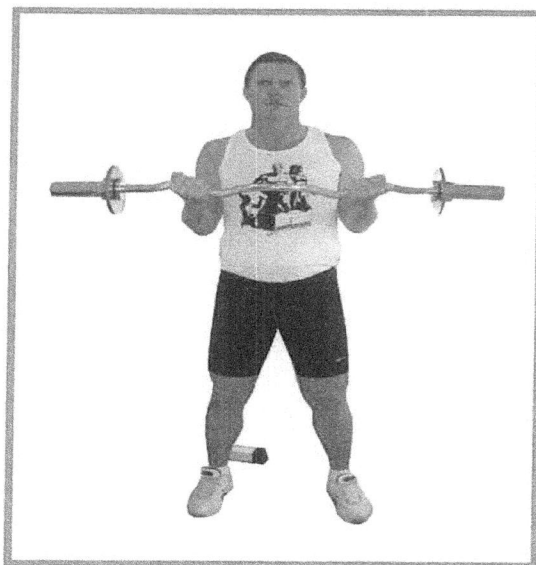

Finish

* Grab bar a little wider than shoulder width- special curl bar should allow palms to turn in slightly, feet about shoulder's width apart, soft knees.
* Keeping elbows down, curl the bar up towards the top of chest.
* Lower it back to start position.

Mike's Special Pointer:
Perhaps the most common mistake on bar curls is to bring the elbows forward at the top of the movement. This takes a lot of stress off the bicep muscle and puts it in the joint- exactly what you don't want when you do curls.

Triceps Extensions: Cable

Target Area: Triceps (back of upper arms)

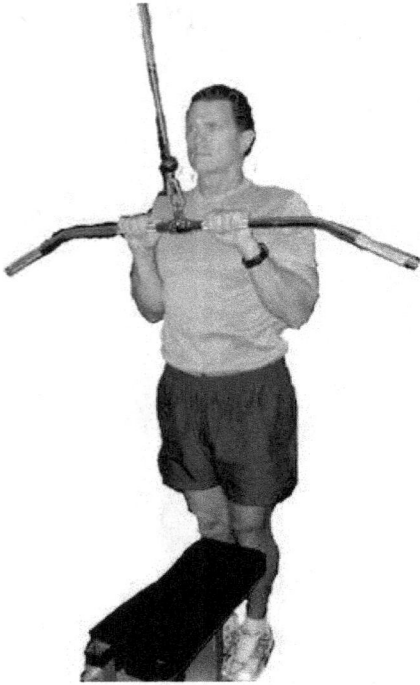

Start

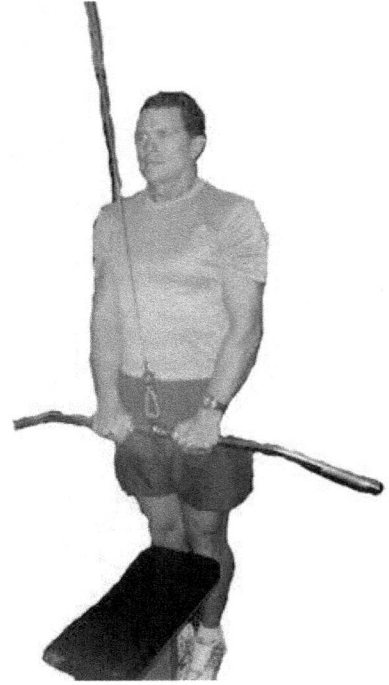

Finish

- Put a straight bar or curved triceps bar on an upper cable machine. Stand straight, knees slightly bent, elbows down, hands in front of shoulders. Push down until arms are fully extended.
- Come back up to the start position.

Mike's Special Pointer:

Keep those elbows in close to your body. They'll want to flare out, but don't let them. Elbows held closer together make for a better triceps workout.

Abdominal Machine

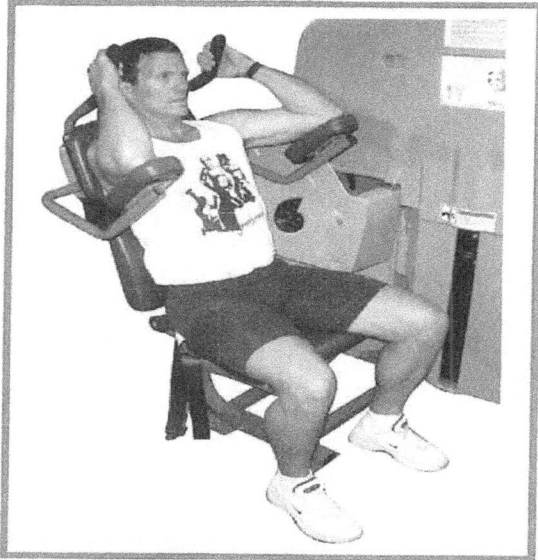

Start

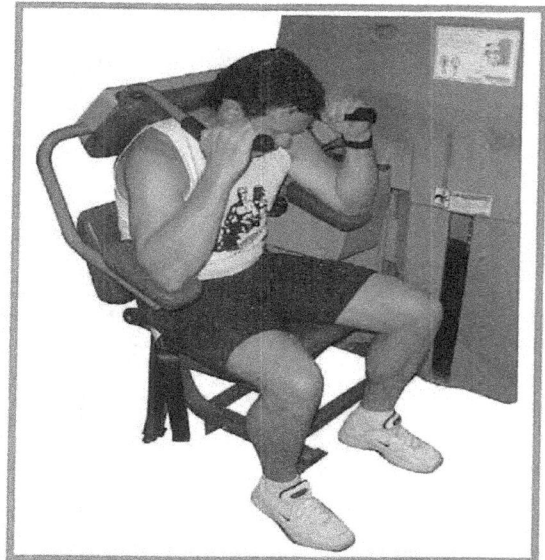

Finish

* Set seat so that your navel is about in line with axis of rotating arm of machine.
* Sit in seat, grab handles (if available), feet flat on floor, sit upright.
* Using your abdominal muscles, pull forward and then down.
* Return to starting position.

Mike's Special Pointer:
Don't allow your back to come out of the seat- keep it back at all times.

Lower Back Machine

TARGET AREA -   Lower Back

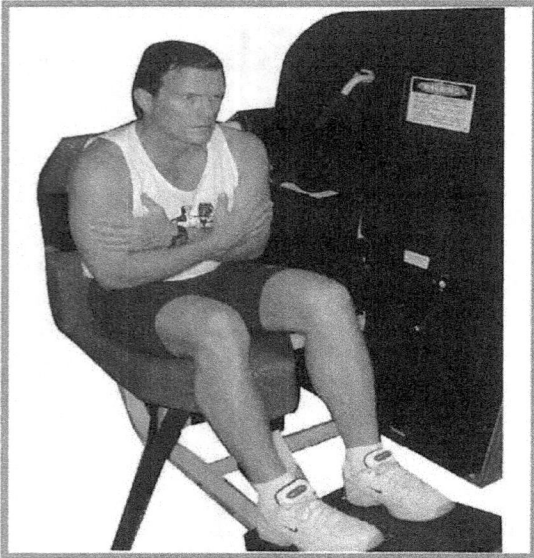

Start

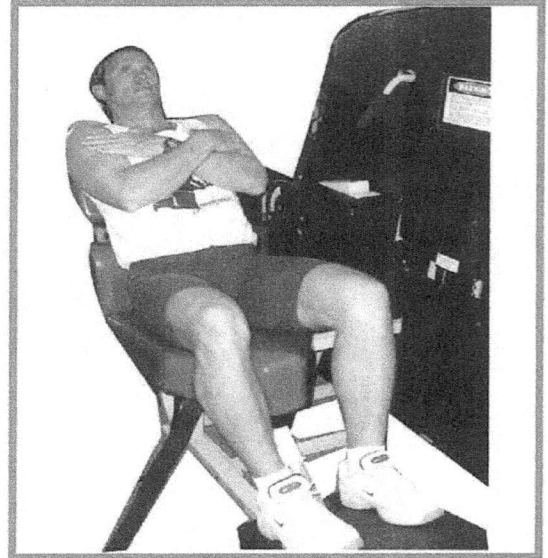

Finish

* Set foot pad so knees are comfortably bent. Sit in machine, cross hands over chest.
* Push back until legs and body are straight or until weight touches at top (depending on which style of machine you use).
* Come forward to a stretch, or until weight touches back down.

Mike's Special Pointer:
Careful on this machine- it's a good exercise, but don't try and lift heavy at first. Start light, and gradually progress as the weeks pass.

Intermediate Male:

Pain Free Functional Strength Workout - Intermediate Male: Quick Sheet – Review and Additional Instructions

Before Starting:

* Be sure you have a way to make small increases when using weights or dumbbells less than 50 pounds.

* Take one workout to get your starting weight established for each exercise. For all exercises, find the weight that you can get one set of 10 reps moderately easy.

* Write down all these starting weights on your *Pain Free Functional Strength* Workout Chart workout chart, just above the word "weight".

* Each exercise is explained in detail in the pages that follow your workout chart.

Pain Free Functional Strength – The Workout

* Your first workout – Do 3 sets of 8 reps for each exercise. (Except for the calf raises, abdominal exercises, shoulder shrugs and wrist curls. Instead of doing 8, 9, 10, 11 and 12 reps you will use 11, 12, 13, 14, and 15 reps for these exercises instead)

* Workout Number 2 – do 3 sets of 9 reps

* Workout Number 3 – do 3 sets of 10 reps

* Workout Number 4 – do 3 sets of 11 reps

* Workout Number 5 – do 3 sets of 12 reps

* Workout Number 6 – Increase the weight by only 5 to 10 percent for each exercise. But now drop your reps back to 3 sets of 8

* Workout Number 7 – do 3 sets of 9 reps

* Workout Number 8 – do 3 sets of 10 reps

* Workout Number 9 – do 3 sets of 11 reps

* Workout Number 10 – do 3 sets of 12 reps

* Workout Number 11 - Increase the weights by 5 to 10 percent once again on those exercises that you got 3 sets of 12 on during the last workout. Continue the normal progression on all the other exercises, or use the next 5 workouts to "even it out" (as described in chapter 6)

* Continue as long as you can using this pattern

* *Pain Free Functional Strength* ends on an exercise when you can no longer get the number of reps that the workout calls for 2 workouts in a row.

*   For the remaining workouts, continue doing those exercises that came to an end for at least your 3 sets of 8 reps, while working the progression for the remaining exercises. When all the exercises have come to their anticipated end, you have finished *Pain Free Functional Strength* – Congratulations!

What now? Pick all new exercises and start back at the beginning. Or continue on this workout but decrease the weight by 1/3rd and do 5, 6, and 7 reps instead of 8 through 12.

Additional exercises and instructions.

1.   Bicycle sit-ups: Do 1 to 2 sets of 15 reps, gradually building up to a total of 50 reps.
2.   Bench knee raises: Do 1 set of 15 reps, build up to 30 or more reps.

Workout Chart - For 8, 9, 10, 11 and 12 reps Intermediate - Male

(Cross off rep counts as you progress through workouts)

Exercise #1: Dumbbell Squats	**Weight:** _____ 8,9,10,11,12 _____ 8,9,10,11,12 _____ 8,9,10,11,12	8,9,10,11,12 8,9,10,11,12 8,9,10,11,12	8,9,10,11,12 8,9,10,11,12 8,9,10,11,12
Exercise #2: Kneeling Leg Curl (2 sets)	**Weight:** _____ 8,9,10,11,12 _____ 8,9,10,11,12 _____ 8,9,10,11,12	8,9,10,11,12 8,9,10,11,12 8,9,10,11,12	8,9,10,11,12 8,9,10,11,12 8,9,10,11,12
Exercise #3: Machine Calf Raise (10,11,12,13,14 reps)	**Weight:** _____ 10,11,12,13,14 _____ 10,11,12,13,14 _____ 10,11,12,13,14	10,11,12,13,14 10,11,12,13,14 10,11,12,13,14	10,11,12,13,14 10,11,12,13,14 10,11,12,13,14
Exercise #4: Bench Press	**Weight:** _____ 8,9,10,11,12 _____ 8,9,10,11,12 _____ 8,9,10,11,12	8,9,10,11,12 8,9,10,11,12 8,9,10,11,12	8,9,10,11,12 8,9,10,11,12 8,9,10,11,12
Exercise #5: 1 Arm Dumbbell Rows	**Weight:** _____ 8,9,10,11,12 _____ 8,9,10,11,12 _____ 8,9,10,11,12	8,9,10,11,12 8,9,10,11,12 8,9,10,11,12	8,9,10,11,12 8,9,10,11,12 8,9,10,11,12
Exercise #6: Dumbbell Lateral Raise	**Weight:** _____ 8,9,10,11,12 _____ 8,9,10,11,12 _____ 8,9,10,11,12	8,9,10,11,12 8,9,10,11,12 8,9,10,11,12	8,9,10,11,12 8,9,10,11,12 8,9,10,11,12
Exercise #7: 1 Arm Conc. Curls	**Weight:** _____ 8,9,10,11,12 _____ 8,9,10,11,12 _____ 8,9,10,11,12	8,9,10,11,12 8,9,10,11,12 8,9,10,11,12	8,9,10,11,12 8,9,10,11,12 8,9,10,11,12
Exercise #8: On Back Bar Triceps Ext.	**Weight:** _____ 8,9,10,11,12 _____ 8,9,10,11,12 _____ 8,9,10,11,12	8,9,10,11,12 8,9,10,11,12 8,9,10,11,12	8,9,10,11,12 8,9,10,11,12 8,9,10,11,12
Exercise #9: Bar Shrugs (10,11,12,13,14 reps)	**Weight:** _____ 10,11,12,13,14 _____ 10,11,12,13,14 _____ 10,11,12,13,14	10,11,12,13,14 10,11,12,13,14 10,11,12,13,14	10,11,12,13,14 10,11,12,13,14 10,11,12,13,14

Exercise #10: Dumbbell Deadlifts	Weight:	8,9,10,11,12		8,9,10,11,12		8,9,10,11,12
		8,9,10,11,12		8,9,10,11,12		8,9,10,11,12
		8,9,10,11,12		8,9,10,11,12		8,9,10,11,12
Exercise #11: Abdominal Machine (10,11,12,13,14 reps)	Weight:	10,11,12,13,14		10,11,12,13,14		10,11,12,13,14
		10,11,12,13,14		10,11,12,13,14		10,11,12,13,14
		10,11,12,13,14		10,11,12,13,14		10,11,12,13,14

Dumbbell Squats

Target Area – Quadriceps and Glutei (front of upper thighs)

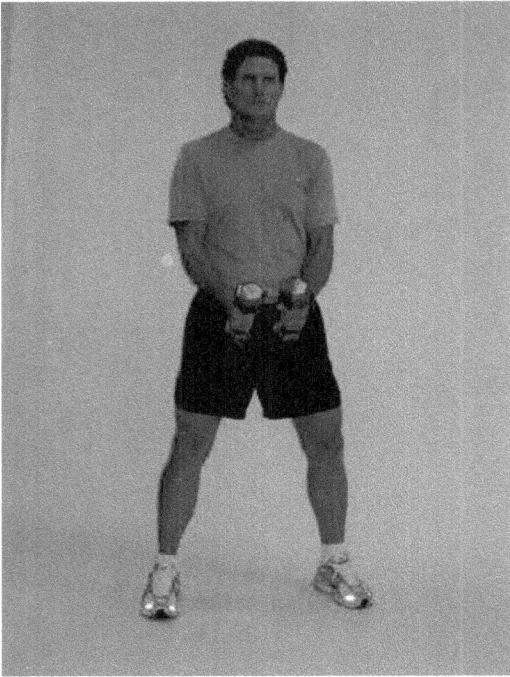

Start

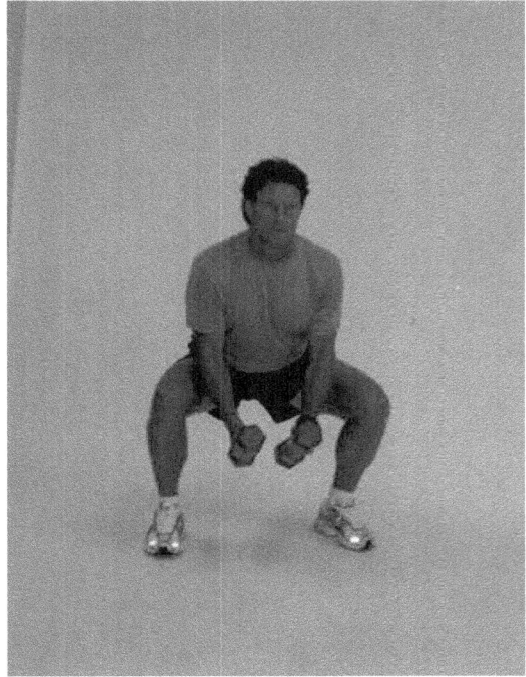

Finish

- Stand with feet at about shoulder's width, toes out slightly.
- Bend down, keeping the back straight, chin up.
- Allow the weights to come down between the knees, or until your upper thighs are close to, or parallel to the ground.
- Push back up to the starting position.

Mike's Special Pointer:

Stay flat footed as you do this exercise. Don't roll back on your heels or go forward on your toes.

Leg Curls - Kneeling

<u>TARGET AREA -</u>   <u>Hamstrings - back of upper legs</u>

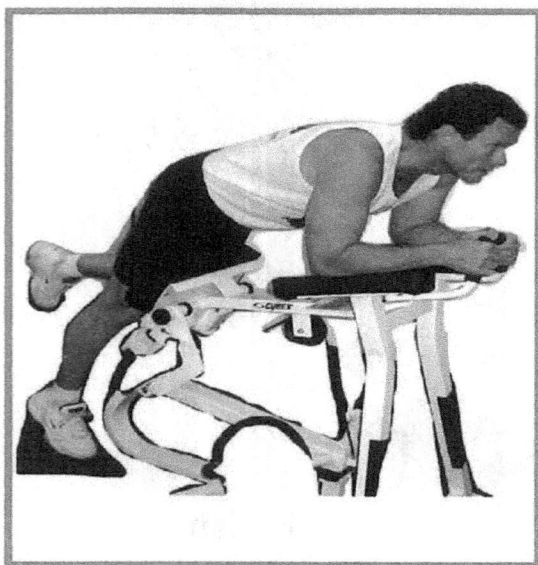

Start

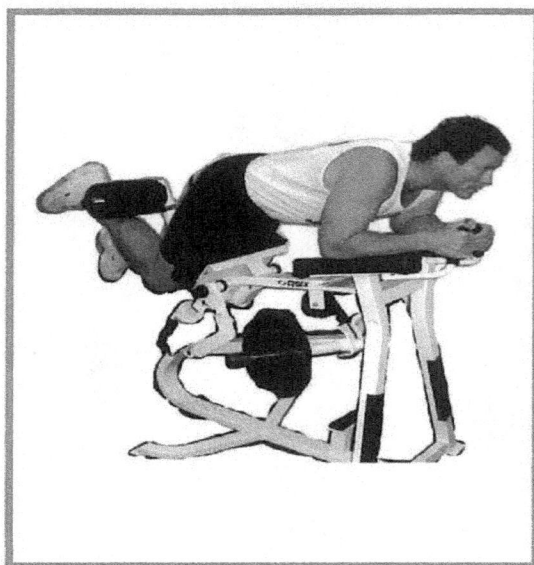

Finish

* Position machine so that you are kneeling on one pad, working ankle behind the lower pad, and upper body resting on forearm pads.
* Look ahead, pull your lower leg up as high as you can, to at least a 90 degree bend of the knee.
* Lower the weight back down until your leg is straight, but be careful not to let the pad go too far, hyper-extending your knee.

Mike's Special Pointer:
This is one of the best hamstring exercises there is, but it's not done very often. It's good for athletes that run in their sport because the exercise more closely mimics the running movement.

Calf Raise Machine - Standing

TARGET AREA -   **Calves - back of lower legs**

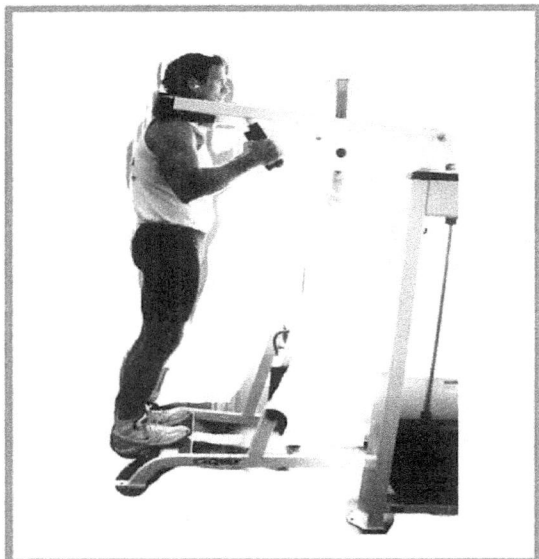

Start

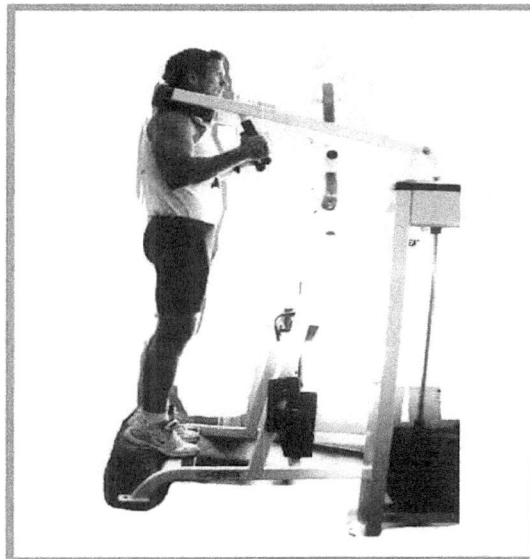

Finish

* Set machine so that you're able to go all the way up and all the way down without the weight stack touching the top or bottom.
* Get under shoulder pads, keep your back straight and lift the weight stack initially by pressing with your legs, not by bending your back.
* Position your feet so that the balls of your feet are on the step, heels hanging over, grab hand grips.
* Allow your calves to stretch fully by bringing your heels as close to the ground as possible, push up onto the balls of your feet as high as possible and pause briefly. Come back to a full stretch.

Mike's Special Pointer:
Keep a very slight bend in your knees while doing this exercise and keep it there for the entire time both up and down. Also, pause at top for at least ½ second for maximum effectiveness.

Bench Press

Target Area – Pectorals (Chest)

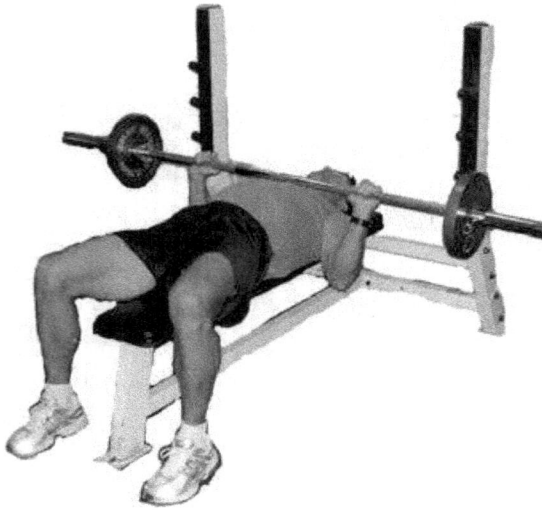 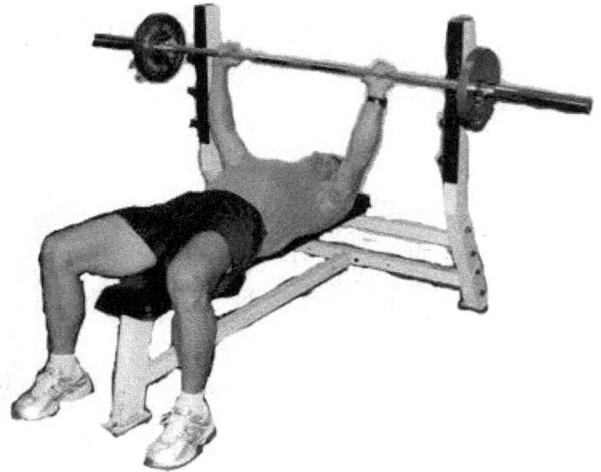

Start   **Finish**

- Lay down flat, grab the bar wider than your shoulders. A good way to know if your arms are spaced correctly is to do a repetition and come down until your upper arms are parallel to the floor. At that position, your forearms should point straight up.
- Lift the bar off the rack and hold it straight up. Lower the bar and bring it slightly forward until you come to a point at, or just below your sternum, (the hard bone at the center of your chest).
- Keep your elbows pointed slightly forward as opposed to being straight back.
- Push up to the starting position.

Mike's Special Pointer:

This is probably the most popular exercise at any given gym, and for good reason – it's a great way to build and firm your chest muscles. But be careful! Don't do a lot of bench presses without balancing your muscles on the other side of your body by doing extra upper back work as well, such as rows.

Dumbbell Rows: One Arm

Target Area – Latissimus (middle and outer back)

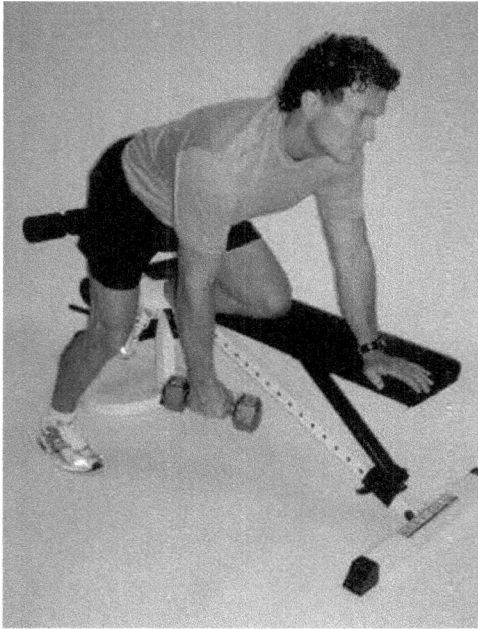

Start

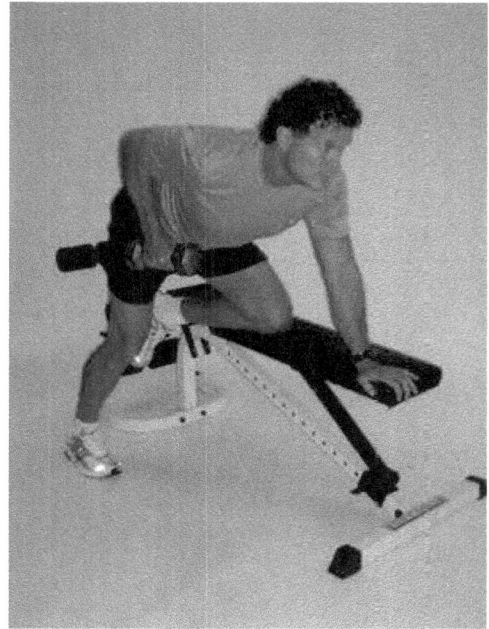

Finish

- On a flat bench, put your knee up for support, (the knee of the leg opposite of the hand that will be doing the exercise).
- Place your other hand down for support.
- Allow the dumbbell to hang in a full stretch.
- Pull the weight up and slightly back so that your hand ends up at your rib cage in the up position.
- Lower the weight to a stretch position, allow your shoulder to drop down slightly for a better stretch.

Mike's Special Pointer:

When you pull up, your forearm should stay approximately straight up and down throughout the exercise. A common mistake is to pull the wrist up under the body so that the forearm angles forward.

Dumbbell Lateral Raises - Standing

TARGET AREA -   Deltoids - shoulders

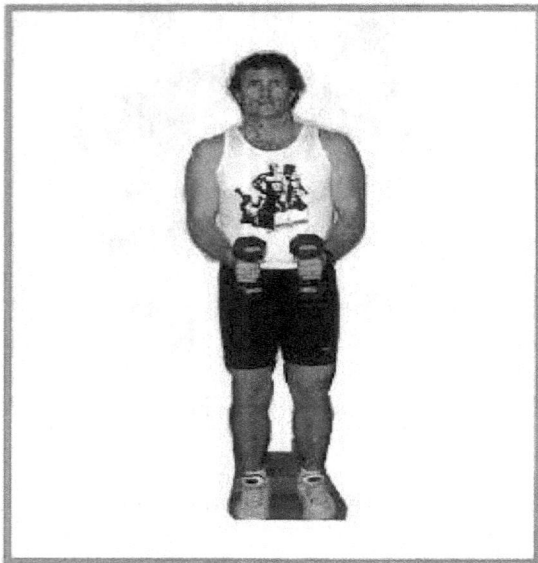

Start

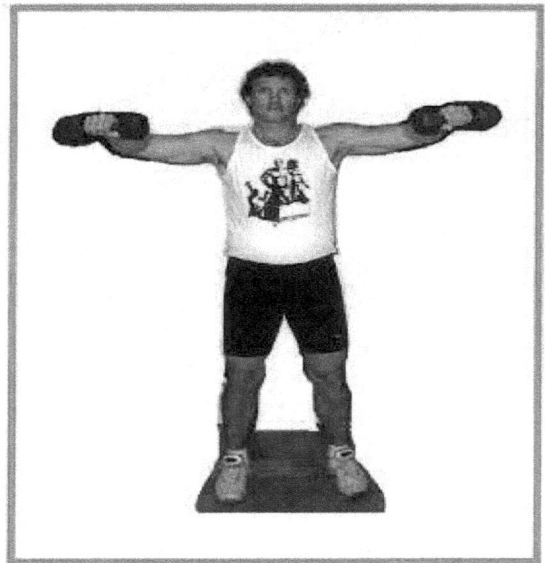

Finish

* Hold dumbbells while standing, palms facing each other, elbows slightly bent, weights approximately at naval height, feet a little more narrow than shoulder's width, knees slightly bent.
* Move dumbbells apart trying to keep the same amount of bend in the elbows
* Come up until your arms are about parallel to the floor; at the top position your forearms should point out slightly as opposed to straight ahead.
* Lower the weights back down keeping the bend in your elbows about the same.

Mike's Special Pointer:
It is not necessary to go higher than parallel to the floor.
That brings in other muscles making the exercise less productive.

Concentration Curls

<u>TARGET AREA -</u>   <u>Biceps - front of upper arms</u>

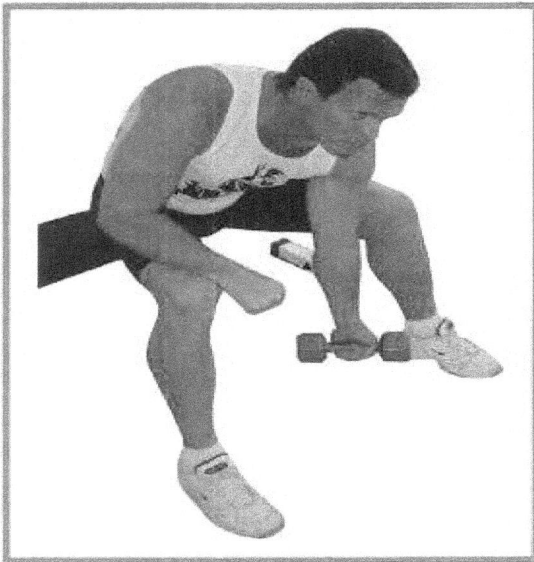

Start

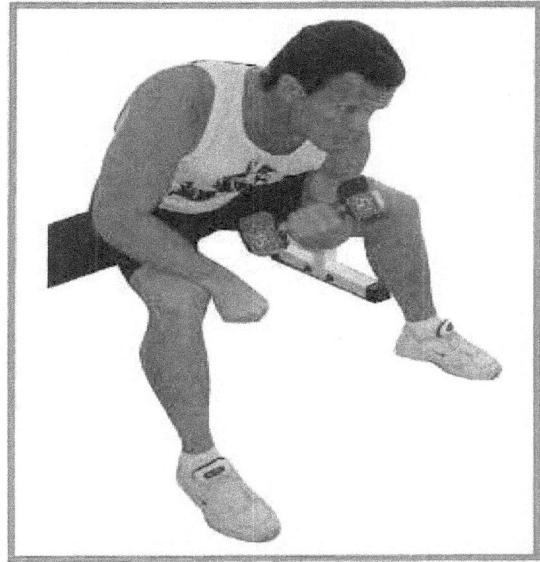

Finish

* Sit sideways on a bench or chair and spread your legs.
* Put non-working arm so that it supports upper body weight just above the knee.
* Hang the working arm down, palm facing towards your other leg, back of upper arm braced against the inside of your leg near your knee.
* Curl the weight up, keeping your upper body steady- go as high as you can.
* Lower the weight back down to start position.

Mike's Special Pointer:
Come all the way down until your arm is straight. Doing bicep curls with a short range of motion can shorten your tendons and make you more prone to injury.

Triceps Extensions: Bar, On Back

Target Area – Triceps (back of upper arms)

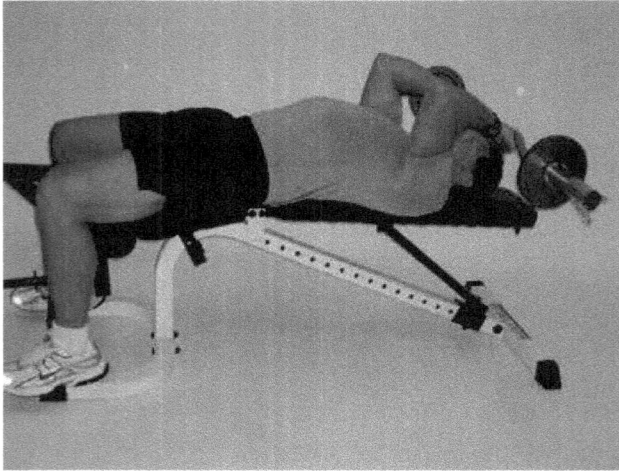

Start

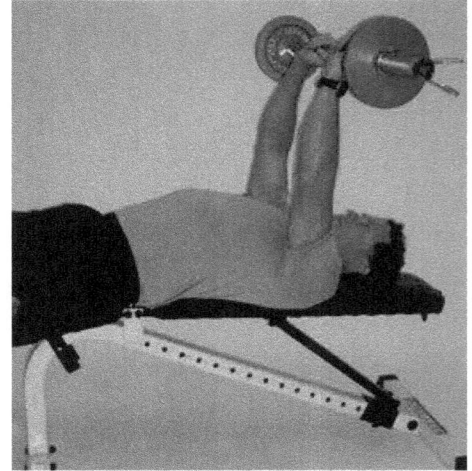

Finish

- Lay flat on your back on a bench, or on the ground, grab the bar narrower than shoulder's width, extend arms so the bar is approximately above your chin.
- Feet up on the bench is optional.
- In a controlled manner, come down, keeping your elbows up.
- Stop the bar just before it reaches your forehead.
- Push back up, keeping your elbows pointed forward, don't lock the elbows out up at the top position.

Mike's Special Pointer:

Be sure to keep your elbows pointed forward, they'll want to push out to the sides, especially when pushing up. Also, be careful to control the weight coming down or you could hit your head with the bar.

Shrugs - Bar

TARGET AREA -   Trapezius - upper back

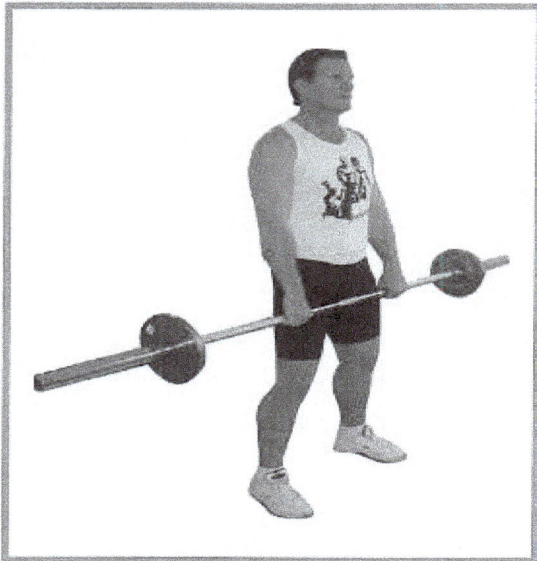

Start

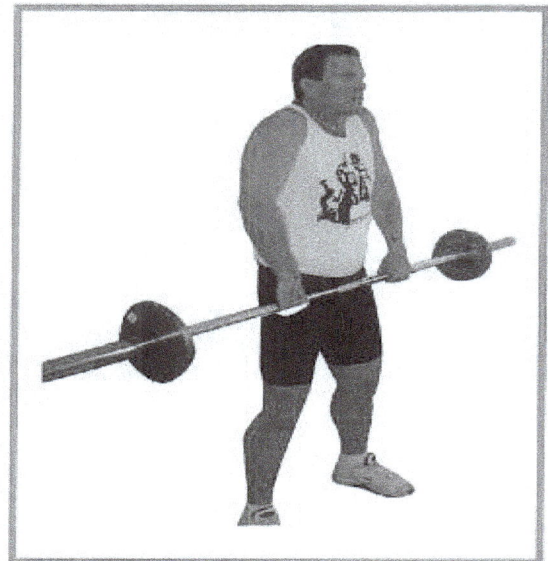

Finish

* Place your feet wider than your shoulders, grab bar at about shoulder's width, palms facing you, keep a soft bend in your knees.
* Shrug your shoulders up as high as you can without hardly any bend in your elbows.
* Come back down and allow the bar to stretch all the way down.

Mike's Special Pointer:
Try pausing at the top for a full count of 2-3 seconds. Shrugs are such a short range movement that this pause seems to really help work the muscles.

Dumbbell Dead Lifts

Target Area – Glutei, (buttocks and lower back)

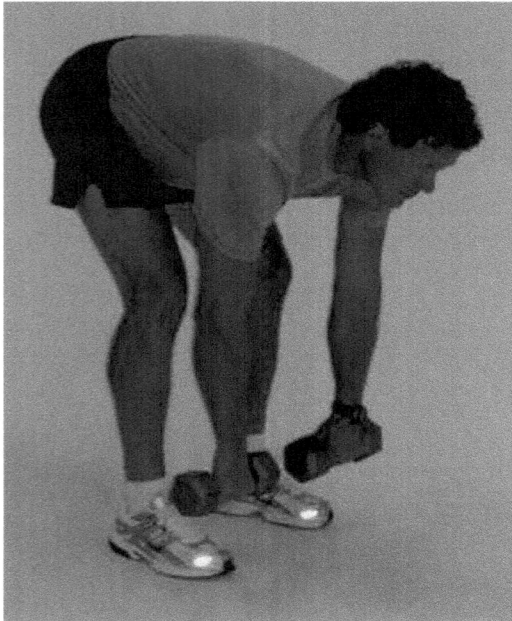

Start

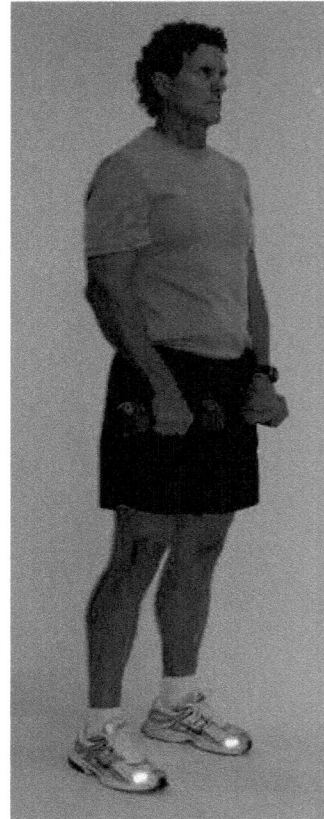

Finish

- Start with feet about shoulder's width, dumbbells at your sides. Bend at the waist and come down until your back is about parallel to the ground.

- As you come down, be sure to keep your back flat, keep your chin up. At the down position, your arms should be hanging straight down. Pull back up to the starting position.

- Come up all the way, but don't lean back at the top.

Mike's Special Pointer:

Be sure to keep your back flat during this exercise, as opposed to rounded. Use a mirror to check your form by standing sideways to the mirror.

Abdominal Machine

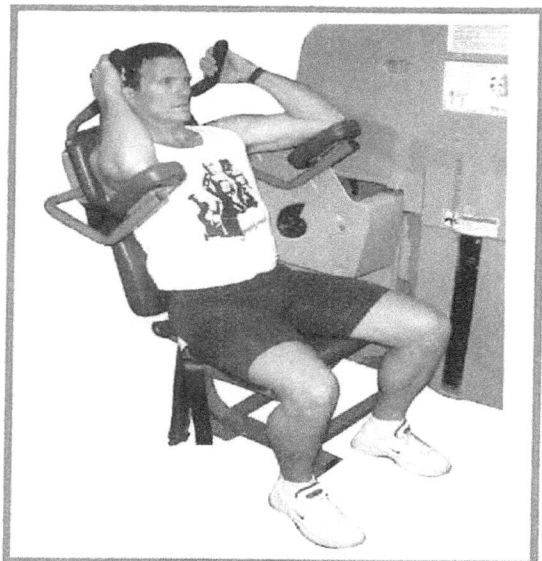

Start

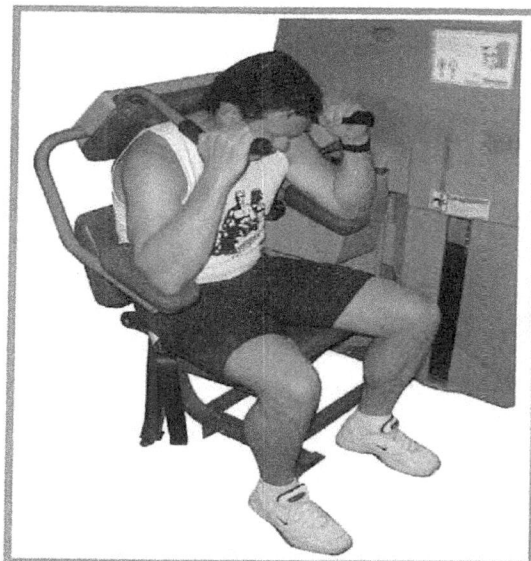

Finish

* Set seat so that your navel is about in line with axis of rotating arm of machine.
* Sit in seat, grab handles (if available), feet flat on floor, sit upright.
* Using your abdominal muscles, pull forward and then down.
* Return to starting position.

Mike's Special Pointer:
Don't allow your back to come out of the seat- keep it back at all times.

100

Sit Ups - Bicycle

TARGET AREA -   Abdominals & Obliques - front & sides of torso

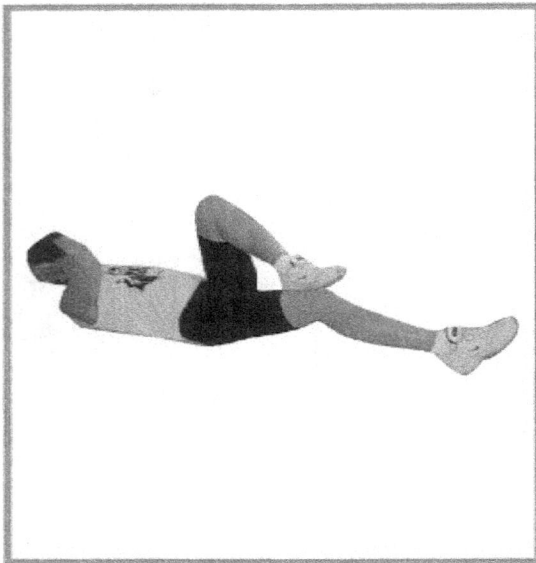

Start

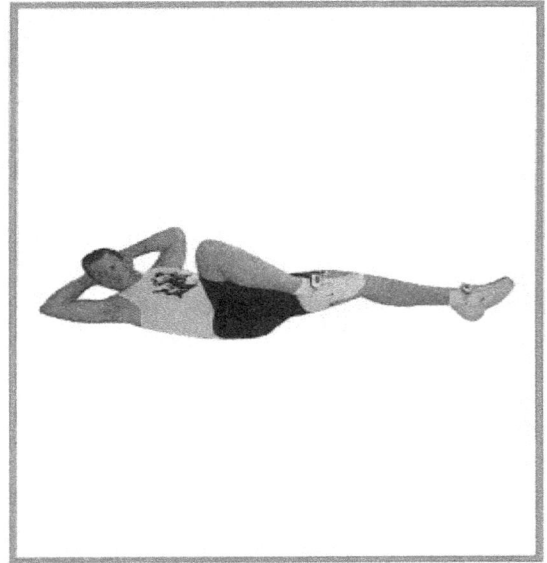

Finish

* Lay flat on your back on the floor or a mat, lightly clasp your fingers behind your head, raise both feet off the floor with knees slightly bent.
* Bring one knee up as the opposite elbow turns toward it.
* Stop well short of the elbow touching the knee.
* Next, bring the other leg in as the original leg extends out.
* While this is happening you're pivoting your upper body the other way so that your other elbow is moving towards your opposite knee.
* Keep crisscrossing until you've done the desired number of repetitions.

Mike's Special Pointer:
Don't swing your shoulders side to side on the floor. Think of a pivot rod attached to the top of your head, not allowing your head to move all around- only pivot. That's the action you're looking for.

Knee Raises: Bench

Target Area – Abdominal (front of torso)

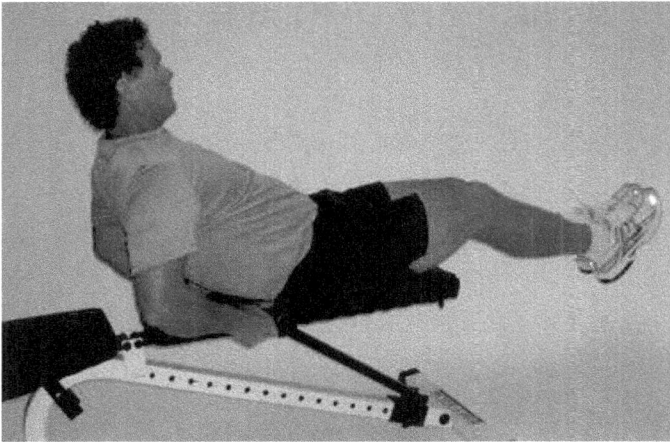

Start

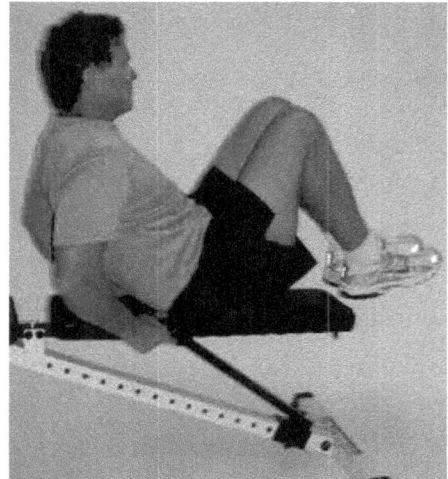

Finish

- Sit on a flat bench, lean back and hold on just behind your buttocks, extend your feet, but do not lock the knees.
- Bring your knees up as you move your upper body slightly forward.
- There should be very little pressure on your hands.
- Extend your legs forward to the start position as you move your upper body back slightly.

Mike's Special Pointer:

Not locking your knees on the extended position is very important. If you lock your knees you greatly increase the risk of injury to your lower back.

Intermediate Female:

Pain Free Functional Strength Workout- Intermediate Female: Quick Sheet – Review and Additional Instructions

Before Starting:

* Be sure you have a way to make small increases when using weights or dumbbells less than 50 pounds.
* Take one workout to get your starting weight established for each exercise. For all exercises, find the weight that you can get one set of 10 reps moderately easy.
* Write down all these starting weights on your *Pain Free Functional Strength* workout chart, just above the word "weight".
* Each exercise is explained in detail in the pages that follow your workout chart.

Pain Free Functional Strength: The Workout

* Your first workout – Do 3 sets of 8 reps for each exercise. (Except for the calf raises, abdominal exercises, shoulder shrugs and wrist curls. Instead of doing 8, 9, 10, 11 and 12 reps you will use 11, 12, 13, 14, and 15 reps for these exercises instead)
* Workout Number 2 – do 3 sets of 9 reps
* Workout Number 3 – do 3 sets of 10 reps
* Workout Number 4 – do 3 sets of 11 reps
* Workout Number 5 – do 3 sets of 12 reps
* Workout Number 6 – Increase the weight by only 5 to 10 percent for each exercise. But now drop your reps back to 3 sets of 8
* Workout Number 7 – do 3 sets of 9 reps
* Workout Number 8 – do 3 sets of 10 reps
* Workout Number 9 – do 3 sets of 11 reps
* Workout Number 10 – do 3 sets of 12 reps
* Workout Number 11 - Increase the weights by 5 to 10 percent once again on those exercises that you got 3 sets of 12 on during the last workout. Continue the normal progression on all the other exercises, or use the next 5 workouts to "even it out" (as described in chapter 6)
* Continue as long as you can using this pattern
* *Pain Free Functional Strength* ends on an exercise when you can no longer get the number of reps that the workout calls for 2 workouts in a row.
* For the remaining workouts, continue doing those exercises that came to an end for at least your 3 sets of 8 reps, while working the progression for the remaining exercises. When all the exercises

have come to their anticipated end, you have finished *Pain Free Functional Strength* – Congratulations!

What now? Pick all new exercises and start back at the beginning. Or continue on this workout but decrease the weight by 1/3rd and do 5, 6, and 7 reps instead of 8 through 12.

Workout Chart - For 8, 9, 10, 11 and 12 reps Intermediate - Female

(Cross off rep counts as you progress through workouts)

Exercise #1: Lunges - Alternating	Weight: _____ 8,9,10,11,12 _____ 8,9,10,11,12 _____ 8,9,10,11,12	_____ 8,9,10,11,12 _____ 8,9,10,11,12	_____ 8,9,10,11,12 _____ 8,9,10,11,12
Exercise #2: Kneeling Leg Curl (2 sets)	Weight: _____ 8,9,10,11,12 _____ 8,9,10,11,12 _____ 8,9,10,11,12	_____ 8,9,10,11,12 _____ 8,9,10,11,12	_____ 8,9,10,11,12 _____ 8,9,10,11,12
Exercise #3: Calf raise Leg Press Machine (10,11,12,13,14 reps)	Weight: _____ 10,11,12,13,14 _____ 10,11,12,13,14 _____ 10,11,12,13,14	_____ 10,11,12,13,14 _____ 10,11,12,13,14	_____ 10,11,12,13,14 _____ 10,11,12,13,14
Exercise #4: Dumbbell Bench Press	Weight: _____ 8,9,10,11,12 _____ 8,9,10,11,12 _____ 8,9,10,11,12	_____ 8,9,10,11,12 _____ 8,9,10,11,12	_____ 8,9,10,11,12 _____ 8,9,10,11,12
Exercise #5: Pull Downs, Front	Weight: _____ 8,9,10,11,12 _____ 8,9,10,11,12 _____ 8,9,10,11,12	_____ 8,9,10,11,12 _____ 8,9,10,11,12	_____ 8,9,10,11,12 _____ 8,9,10,11,12
Exercise #6: Dumbbell Military Press Seated	Weight: _____ 8,9,10,11,12 _____ 8,9,10,11,12 _____ 8,9,10,11,12	_____ 8,9,10,11,12 _____ 8,9,10,11,12	_____ 8,9,10,11,12 _____ 8,9,10,11,12
Exercise #7: Dumbbell Curls, Alt. Standing	Weight: _____ 8,9,10,11,12 _____ 8,9,10,11,12 _____ 8,9,10,11,12	_____ 8,9,10,11,12 _____ 8,9,10,11,12	_____ 8,9,10,11,12 _____ 8,9,10,11,12
Exercise #8: Dumbbell Triceps Ext. On Back	Weight: _____ 8,9,10,11,12 _____ 8,9,10,11,12 _____ 8,9,10,11,12	_____ 8,9,10,11,12 _____ 8,9,10,11,12	_____ 8,9,10,11,12 _____ 8,9,10,11,12
Exercise #9: Dumbbell Shrugs (10,11,12,13,14 reps)	Weight: _____ 10,11,12,13,14 _____ 10,11,12,13,14 _____ 10,11,12,13,14	_____ 10,11,12,13,14 _____ 10,11,12,13,14	_____ 10,11,12,13,14 _____ 10,11,12,13,14

Exercise #10: Dumbbell Deadlifts	Weight:	8,9,10,11,12		8,9,10,11,12		8,9,10,11,12
		8,9,10,11,12		8,9,10,11,12		8,9,10,11,12
		8,9,10,11,12		8,9,10,11,12		8,9,10,11,12

Additional exercises and instructions.

1. Crunches - Do 1 to 2 sets of 15 reps, gradually building up to a total of 50 reps.

2. Bench knee raises - Do 1 to 2 sets of 15 reps, gradually building up to a total of 30 reps

3. Bicycle Sit Ups - Do 1 set of 15 reps, build up to 30 or more reps.

Lunges: Alternating

Target Area – Quadriceps and Glutei (front of upper legs and buttocks)

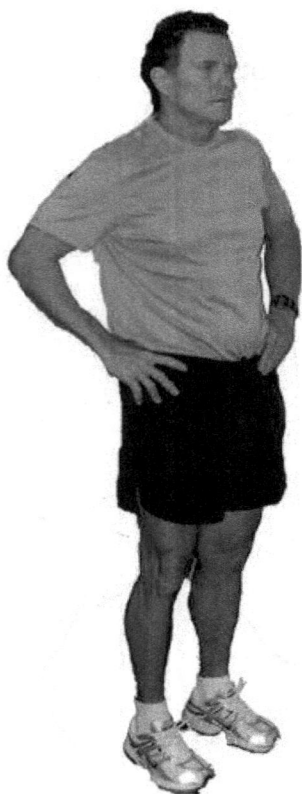

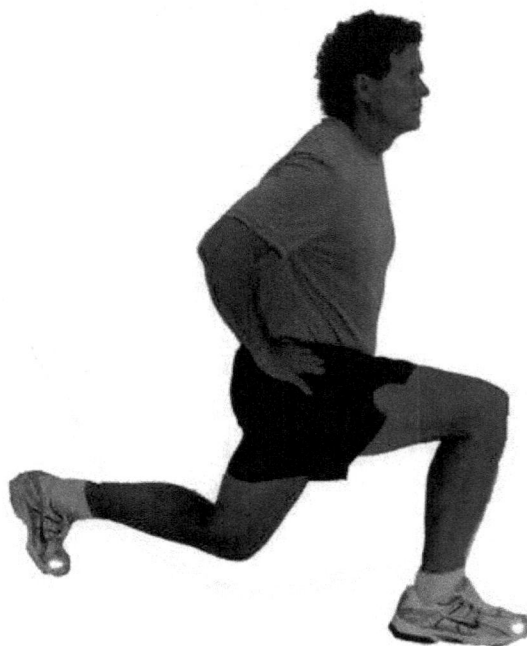

Start   **Finish**

- With your feet together, start with hands on hips, or holding dumbbells if needed.
- Step forward with one leg far enough forward that you feel a stretch in the back leg.
- Go down with the forward leg until the back knee almost touches the ground.
- Push with the forward leg and continue back to the start position (with your feet next to each other). Next, do the other leg in an alternating fashion.

Mike's Special Pointer:

When doing lunges, be sure your forward knee does not go in front of your foot. Notice in the picture that the knee is above the toes. This is a safeguard against knee injury.

Leg Curls - Kneeling

TARGET AREA -   Hamstrings - back of upper legs

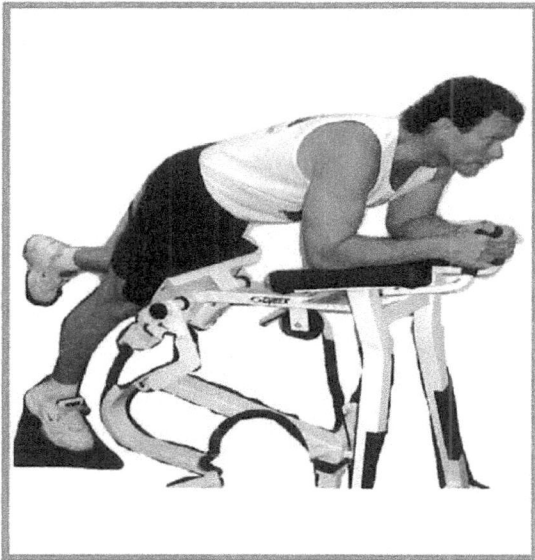

Start

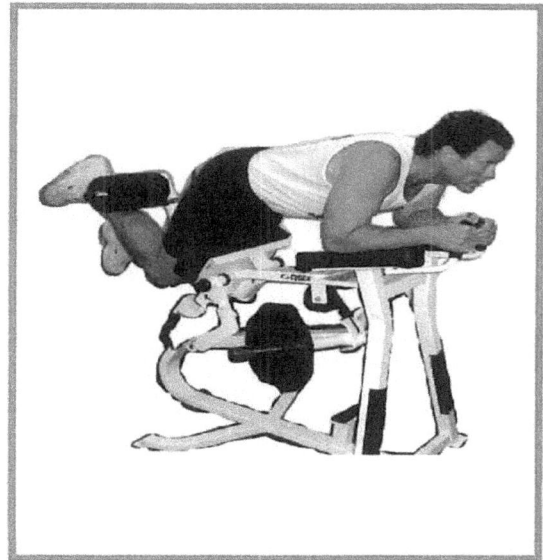

Finish

* Position machine so that you are kneeling on one pad, working ankle behind the lower pad, and upper body resting on forearm pads.
* Look ahead, pull your lower leg up as high as you can, to at least a 90 degree bend of the knee.
* Lower the weight back down until your leg is straight, but be careful not to let the pad go too far, hyper-extending your knee.

Mike's Special Pointer:
This is one of the best hamstring exercises there is, but it's not done very often. It's good for athletes that run in their sport because the exercise more closely mimics the running movement.

Calf Raises - Leg Press Machine

TARGET AREA -   Calves - back of lower legs

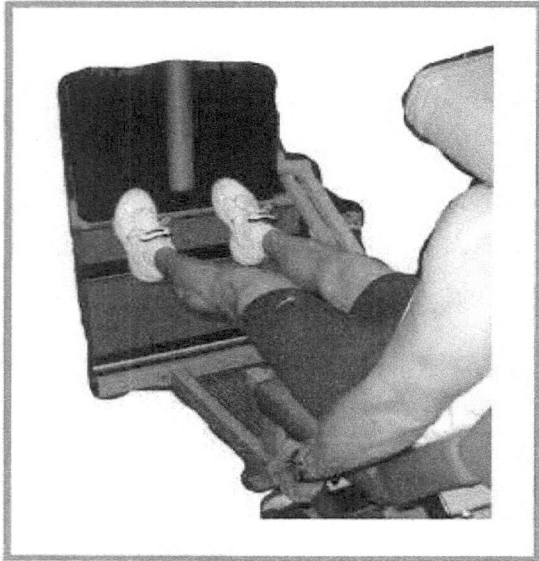

Start

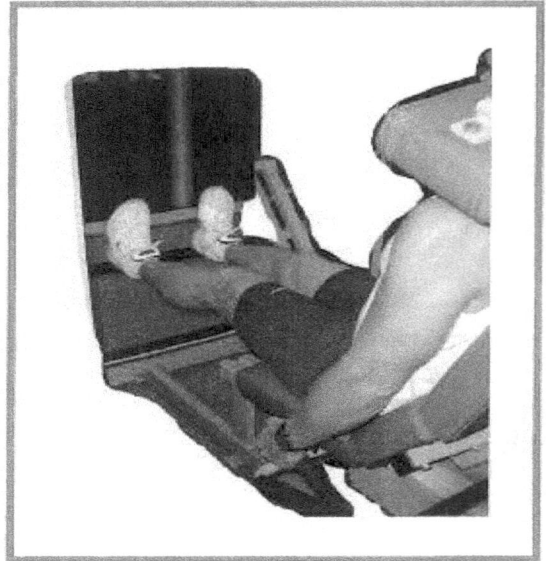

Finish

* Use a standard leg press machine, but be sure it is compatible for doing calf raises.
* Set the seat position so you can do a full range of motion on the calf raise without the weight touching back down after each repetition.
* Place your feet so that the upper 1/3 of your feet are on the foot pad.
* Push your toes forward as if you are trying to stand on your toes.
* Next, bring your toes back towards you until you feel a good stretch.
* Your knees should be only slightly bent the whole time.

Mike's Special Pointer:
You may need to readjust your feet every 3 or 4 repetitions - they tend to slide down as you do this exercise.

Dumbbell Bench Press

Target Area – Pectorals (chest)

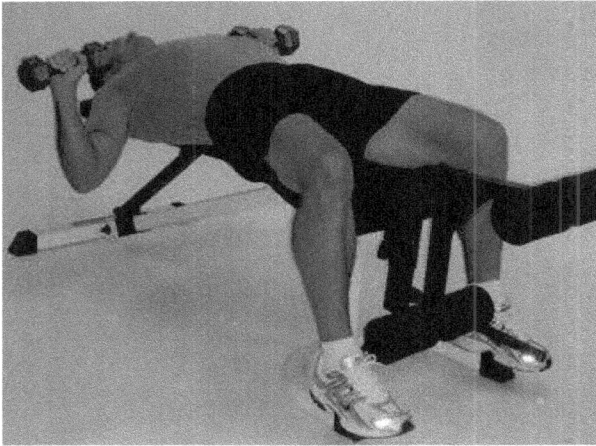

Start

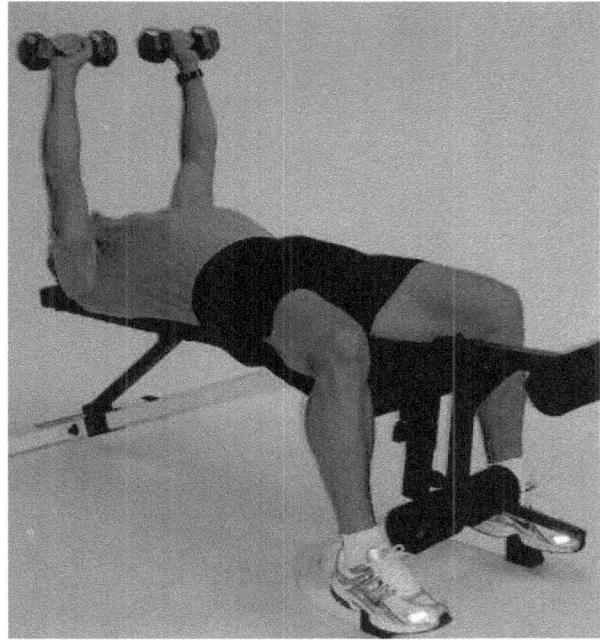

Finish

- Lay flat on your back, putting your feet up is optional.
- Start with the weights wider than your shoulders, elbows at or slightly below the bench.
- Push up and allow the weights to come close together at the top without touching.
- Don't lock out your elbows at the top.
- Come back down to the start position, but don't let your forearms angle out – keep them straight up.

Mike's Special Pointer:

When pushing up, it's OK if your elbows are slightly forward. Many people can develop shoulder injuries if they try and force their elbows way back while doing the exercise.

Pull Downs: Front

Target Area – Latissimus (middle and outer back)

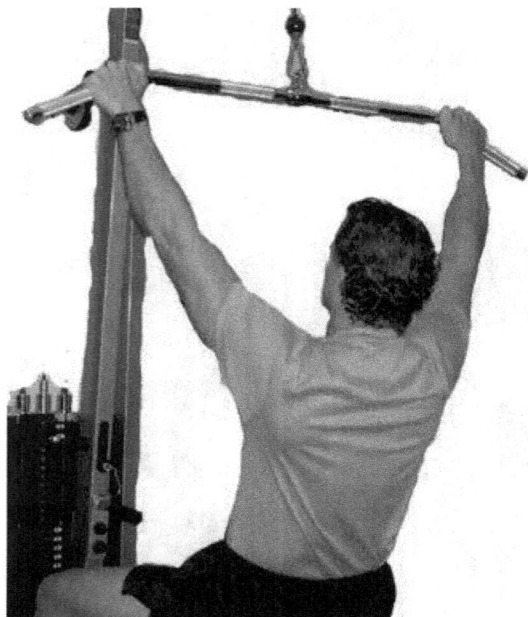 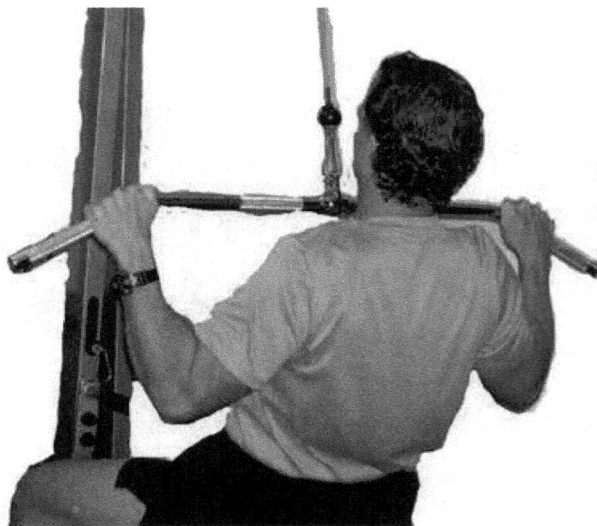

Start   **Finish**

- Position hands wider than your shoulders, palms facing out forward, away from you.
- Pull straight down until the bar comes at or below your chin.
- Raise the bar back up to the starting position, be sure your arms are fully extended giving you a full stretch.

Mike's Special Pointer:

When coming down, don't turn your forearms down so that your palms angle down. When in the finish position, your palms should be facing straight ahead.

Dumbbell Military Press: Seated

Target Area – Deltoids (shoulders)

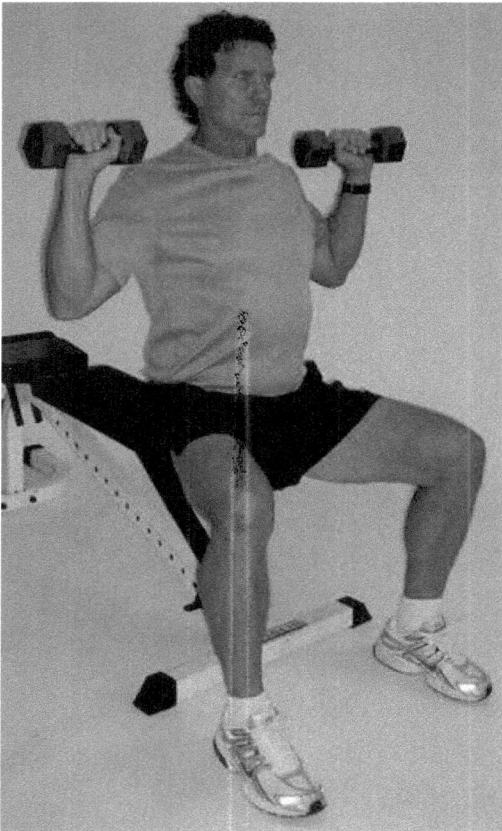

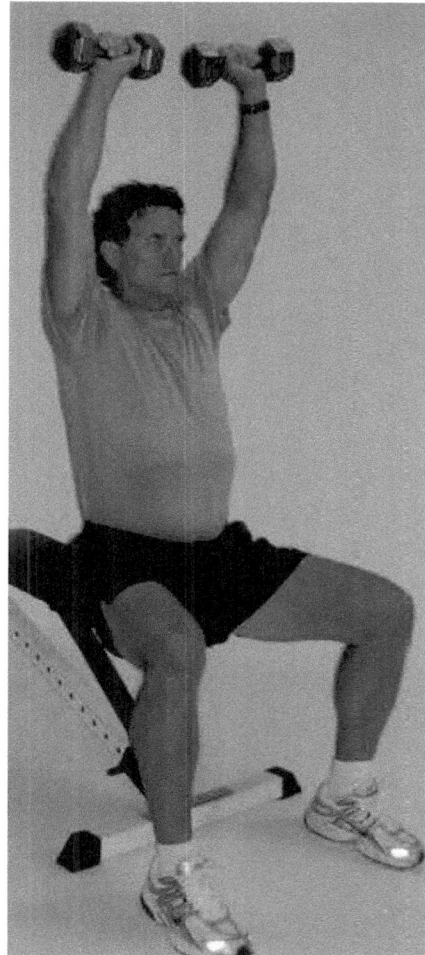

Start   **Finish**

- Hold the dumbbells just wider than your shoulders, with the weights parallel to the floor.
- Push the weights up, and the hands will naturally come closer to each other as you get higher and higher.
- Raise the weights until the elbows are just short of locking out.
- Lower the weights back down to the start position.

Mike's Special Pointer:

Make sure your back is supported by the back rest if the bench you are using has one. Keep your head and neck relaxed as you push the weight over your head.

Dumbbell Curls: Alternating, Standing

Target Area – Biceps (front of upper arms)

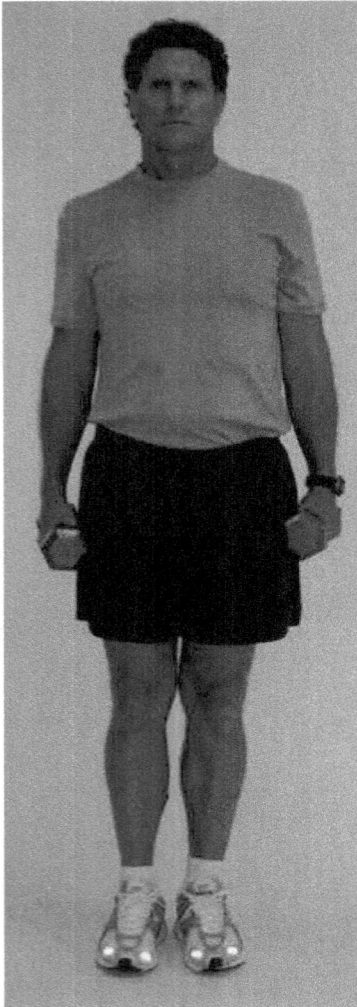

Start

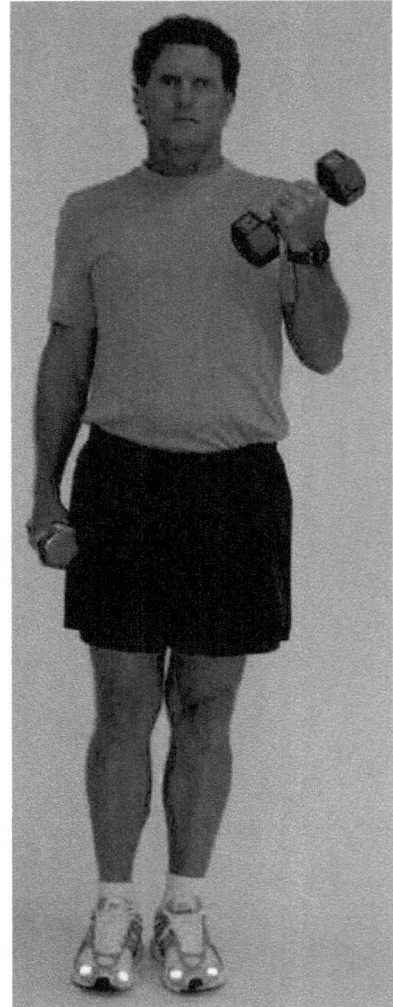

Finish

- Stand with feet slightly apart, knees softly bent, arms hanging at side with palms in.
- Curl one arm up, turn it as you come up, so palm faces back at top.
- Lower back down to full extension, twisting back to the way you started.
- Alternate hands until you reach the desired number of reps.

Mike's Special Pointer:

The hands and forearms will often tire before the biceps give out. Although not common practice, using wrist straps on this exercise may help you to work your biceps harder.

Dumbbell Triceps Extension: On Back

Target Area – Triceps (back of upper arms)

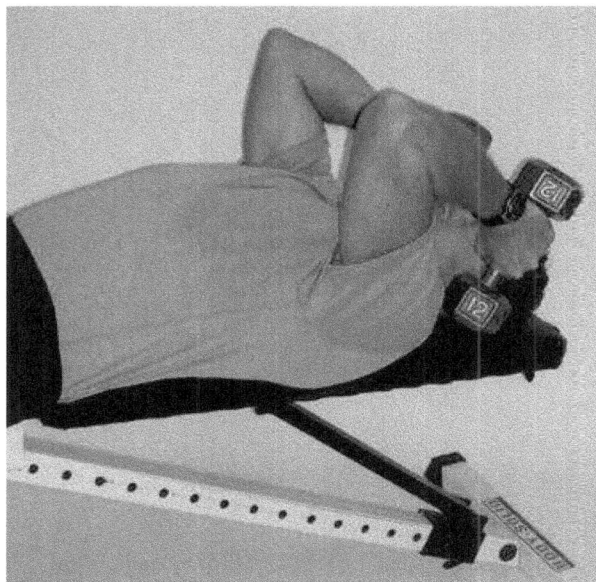

Start

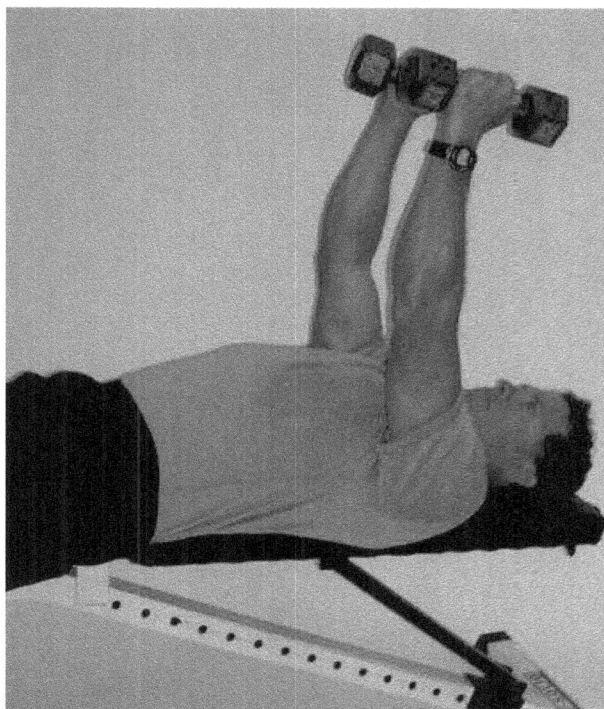

Finish

- Lay flat on a bench, knees up or down according to your preference, dumbbells held straight up, palms facing towards each other.
- Keeping elbows in and up, lower the weights so your hands come approximately to your ears.
- Push back up to the start position.

Mike's Special Pointer:

Keep those elbows in the same place. They tend to want to move backwards and forwards as you do the movements. Don't let that happen though – keep them stationary.

Dumbbell Shrugs

Target Area: Trapezius (upper back)

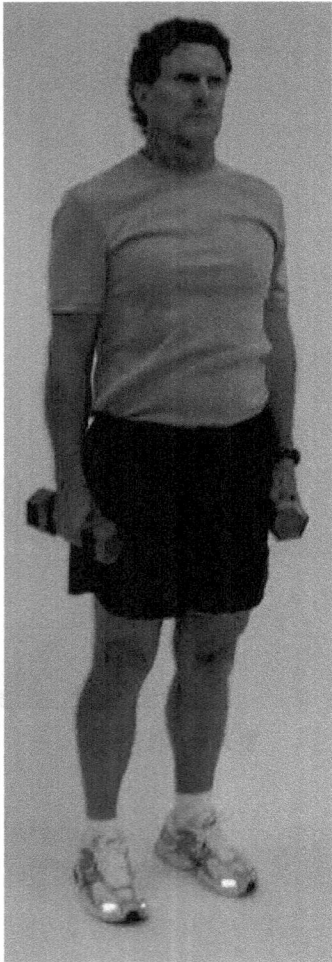

Start

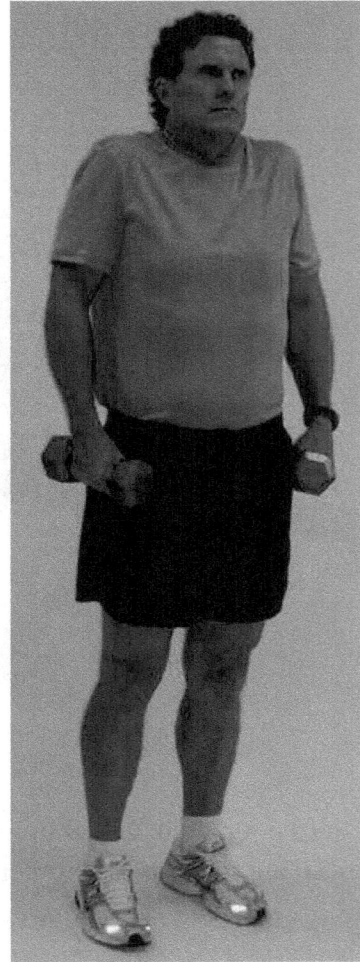

Finish

- Stand holding dumbbells at your sides, feet close together, knees slightly bent, palms facing in.
- Shrug your shoulders up as high as you can with hardly any bend of the elbows.
- Come back down to a full stretch at the bottom.

Mike's Special Pointer:

Dumbbell shrugs have one advantage over regular bar shrugs. You can move the weight forward or backwards a little until you feel it the best, whereas the bar only allows you one angle.

Dumbbell Dead Lifts

Target Area – Glutei, (buttocks and lower back)

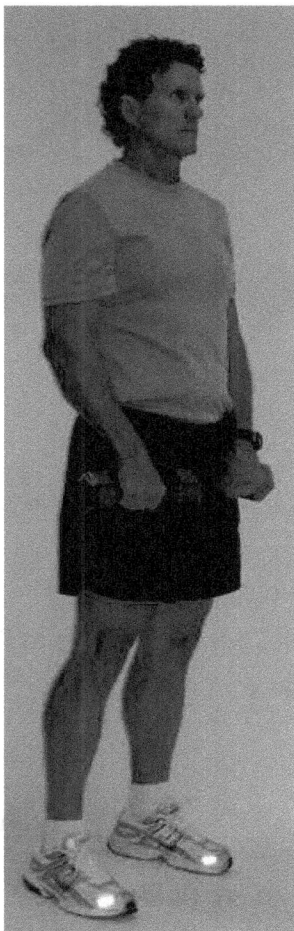

Start

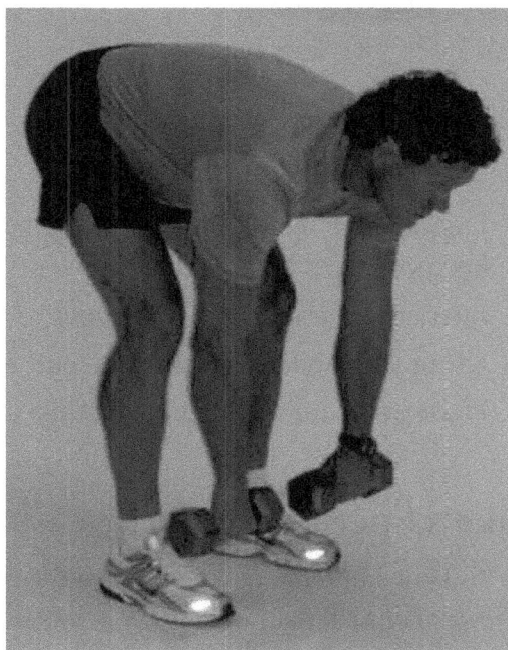

Finish

- Start with feet about shoulder's width, dumbbells at your sides. Bend at the waist and come down until your back is about parallel to the ground.
- As you come down, be sure to keep your back flat, keep your chin up. At the down position, your arms should be hanging straight down. Pull back up to the starting position.
- Come up all the way, but don't lean back at the top.

Mike's Special Pointer:

Be sure to keep your back flat during this exercise, as opposed to rounded. Use a mirror to check your form by standing sideways to the mirror.

Crunches

Target Area – Abdominals (front of torso)

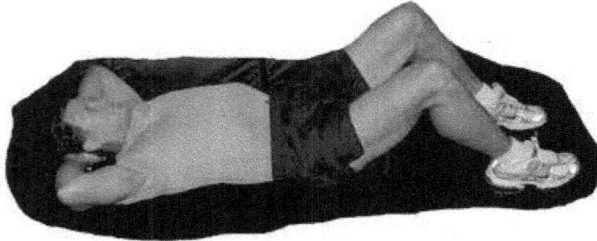 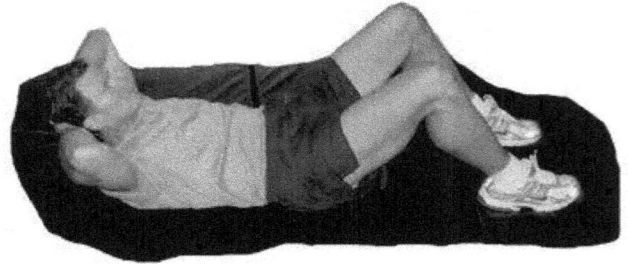

Start **Finish**

- Lay flat on a mat or the floor, keep your lower back pressed down against the floor, raise knees but keep your feet flat on the floor.
- Interlace your fingers behind your head, point your elbows mostly out to the sides.
- Using your abdominal muscles, curl up as you press your lower back further down into the floor.
- Pause at the top for a moment at the top, and then return back to the start position.

Mike's Special Pointer:

How high you come up when doing crunches makes a big difference on the effectiveness of the exercise. Try to actually get your shoulder blades up off the floor when in the finish position.

Knee Raises: Bench

Target Area – Abdominal (front of torso)

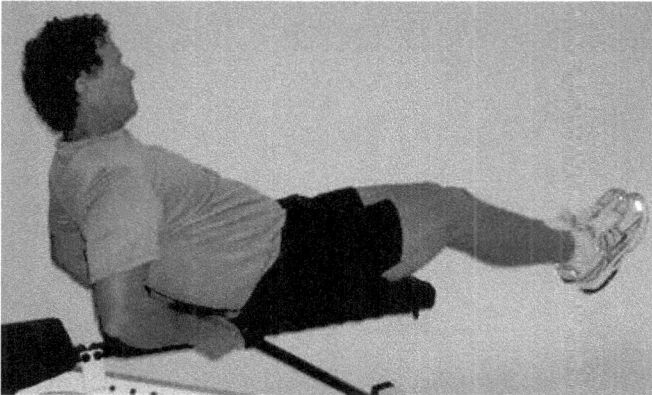

Start

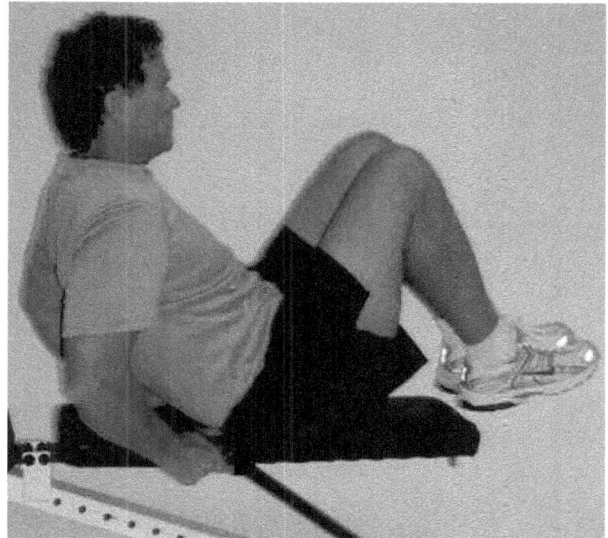

Finish

- Sit on a flat bench, lean back and hold on just behind your buttocks, extend your feet, but do not lock the knees.
- Bring your knees up as you move your upper body slightly forward.
- There should be very little pressure on your hands.
- Extend your legs forward to the start position as you move your upper body back slightly.

Mike's Special Pointer:

Not locking your knees on the extended position is very important. If you lock your knees you greatly increase the risk of injury to your lower back.

Sit Ups - Bicycle

<u>TARGET AREA -</u>   <u>Abdominals & Obliques - front & sides of torso</u>

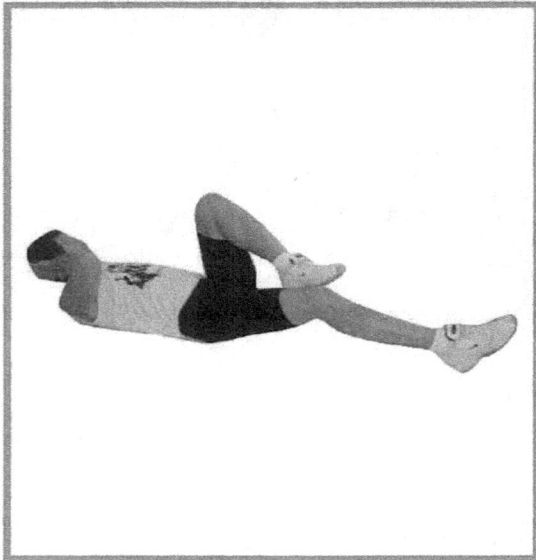

Start

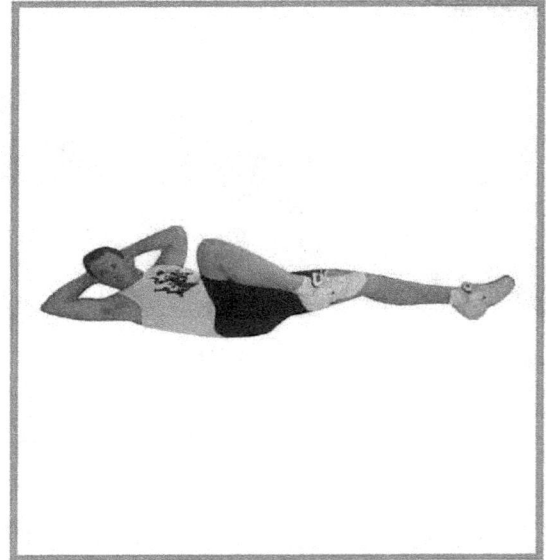

Finish

* Lay flat on your back on the floor or a mat, lightly clasp your fingers behind your head, raise both feet off the floor with knees slightly bent.
* Bring one knee up as the opposite elbow turns toward it.
* Stop well short of the elbow touching the knee.
* Next, bring the other leg in as the original leg extends out.
* While this is happening you're pivoting your upper body the other way so that your other elbow is moving towards your opposite knee.
* Keep crisscrossing until you've done the desired number of repetitions.

Mike's Special Pointer:
Don't swing your shoulders side to side on the floor. Think of a pivot rod attached to the top of your head, not allowing your head to move all around- only pivot. That's the action you're looking for.

Advanced Male:

Pain Free Functional Strength Workout - Advanced Male: Legs, Upper and Lower Back, Biceps

Quick Sheet – Review and Additional Instructions

Before Starting:

* Be sure you have a way to make small increases when using weights or dumbbells less than 50 pounds.

* Take one workout to get your starting weight established for each exercise. For all exercises, find the weight that you can get one set of 10 reps moderately easy.

* Write down all these starting weights on your *Pain Free Functional Strength* workout chart, just above the word "weight".

* Each exercise is explained in detail in the pages that follow your workout chart.

Pain Free Functional Strength: The Workout

* Your first workout – Do 3 sets of 8 reps for each exercise. (Except for the calf raises, abdominal exercises, shoulder shrugs and wrist curls. Instead of doing 8, 9, 10, 11 and 12 reps you will use 11, 12, 13, 14, and 15 reps for these exercises instead)

* Workout Number 2 – do 3 sets of 9 reps

* Workout Number 3 – do 3 sets of 10 reps

* Workout Number 4 – do 3 sets of 11 reps

* Workout Number 5 – do 3 sets of 12 reps

* Workout Number 6 – Increase the weight by only 5 to 10 percent for each exercise. But now drop your reps back to 3 sets of 8

* Workout Number 7 – do 3 sets of 9 reps

* Workout Number 8 – do 3 sets of 10 reps

* Workout Number 9 – do 3 sets of 11 reps

* Workout Number 10 – do 3 sets of 12 reps

* Workout Number 11 - Increase the weights by 5 to 10 percent once again on those exercises that you got 3 sets of 12 on during the last workout. Continue the normal progression on all the other exercises, or use the next 5 workouts to "even it out" (as described in chapter 6)

* Continue as long as you can using this pattern

* *Pain Free Functional Strength* ends on an exercise when you can no longer get the number of reps that the workout calls for 2 workouts in a row.

*   For the remaining workouts, continue doing those exercises that came to an end for at least your 3 sets of 8 reps, while working the progression for the remaining exercises. When all the exercises have come to their anticipated end, you have finished *Pain Free Functional Strength* – Congratulations!

What now? Pick all new exercises and start back at the beginning. Or continue on this workout but decrease the weight by 25-33% and do 5, 6, and 7 reps instead of 8 through 12.

Additional Instructions:

This is one of 2 workouts for the advanced male. Do this work out 2 or 3 days per week, alternating it with the other. Your week will look something like this: Monday and Thursday the legs, lats and biceps workout, Tuesday and Friday the chest, shoulders and abs workout. Rest Wednesday, Saturday and Sunday. Or you could also do the first workout on Monday, Wednesday and Friday and the second Tuesday, Thursday and Saturday, rest Sunday.

Workout Chart - For 8, 9, 10, 11 and 12 reps – Advanced Male: Legs, Upper and Lower Back, Biceps

(Cross off rep counts as you progress through workouts)

Exercise #1: Dead Lift Squats	**Weight:**	8,9,10,11,12		8,9,10,11,12		8,9,10,11,12
		8,9,10,11,12		8,9,10,11,12		8,9,10,11,12
		8,9,10,11,12		8,9,10,11,12		8,9,10,11,12
Exercise #2: Dumbbell Rows, 1 Arm	**Weight:**	8,9,10,11,12		8,9,10,11,12		8,9,10,11,12
		8,9,10,11,12		8,9,10,11,12		8,9,10,11,12
		8,9,10,11,12		8,9,10,11,12		8,9,10,11,12
Exercise #3: Bicep Curls, Bar, Regular Grip	**Weight:**	8,9,10,11,12		8,9,10,11,12		8,9,10,11,12
		8,9,10,11,12		8,9,10,11,12		8,9,10,11,12
		8,9,10,11,12		8,9,10,11,12		8,9,10,11,12
Exercise #4: Leg Curls, Kneeling	**Weight:**	8,9,10,11,12		8,9,10,11,12		8,9,10,11,12
		8,9,10,11,12		8,9,10,11,12		8,9,10,11,12
		8,9,10,11,12		8,9,10,11,12		8,9,10,11,12
Exercise #5: Smith Machine Calf Raises (10,11,12,13,14 reps)	**Weight:**	10,11,12,13,14		10,11,12,13,14		10,11,12,13,14
		10,11,12,13,14		10,11,12,13,14		10,11,12,13,14
		10,11,12,13,14		10,11,12,13,14		10,11,12,13,14
Exercise #6: Pull Downs, Front	**Weight:**	8,9,10,11,12		8,9,10,11,12		8,9,10,11,12
		8,9,10,11,12		8,9,10,11,12		8,9,10,11,12
		8,9,10,11,12		8,9,10,11,12		8,9,10,11,12
Exercise #7: Leg Extensions	**Weight:**	8,9,10,11,12		8,9,10,11,12		8,9,10,11,12
		8,9,10,11,12		8,9,10,11,12		8,9,10,11,12
		8,9,10,11,12		8,9,10,11,12		8,9,10,11,12
Exercise #8: Concentration Curls	**Weight:**	8,9,10,11,12		8,9,10,11,12		8,9,10,11,12
		8,9,10,11,12		8,9,10,11,12		8,9,10,11,12
		8,9,10,11,12		8,9,10,11,12		8,9,10,11,12
Exercise #9: Calf Raise – Reverse (10,11,12,13,14 reps)	**Weight:**	10,11,12,13,14		10,11,12,13,14		10,11,12,13,14
		10,11,12,13,14		10,11,12,13,14		10,11,12,13,14
		10,11,12,13,14		10,11,12,13,14		10,11,12,13,14

Exercise #10: Inner Thigh Machine (Do 2 sets only)	**Weight:**	8,9,10,11,12		8,9,10,11,12		8,9,10,11,12
		8,9,10,11,12		8,9,10,11,12		8,9,10,11,12
		8,9,10,11,12		8,9,10,11,12		8,9,10,11,12
Exercise #11: Outer Thigh Machine (Do 2 sets only)	**Weight:**	8,9,10,11,12		8,9,10,11,12		8,9,10,11,12
		8,9,10,11,12		8,9,10,11,12		8,9,10,11,12
		8,9,10,11,12		8,9,10,11,12		8,9,10,11,12
Exercise #12: Dumbbell Low Back Lifts	**Weight:**	8,9,10,11,12		8,9,10,11,12		8,9,10,11,12
		8,9,10,11,12		8,9,10,11,12		8,9,10,11,12
		8,9,10,11,12		8,9,10,11,12		8,9,10,11,12

Dead Lift Squats

TARGET AREA - Quadriceps & Gluteals - front of upper legs & buttocks

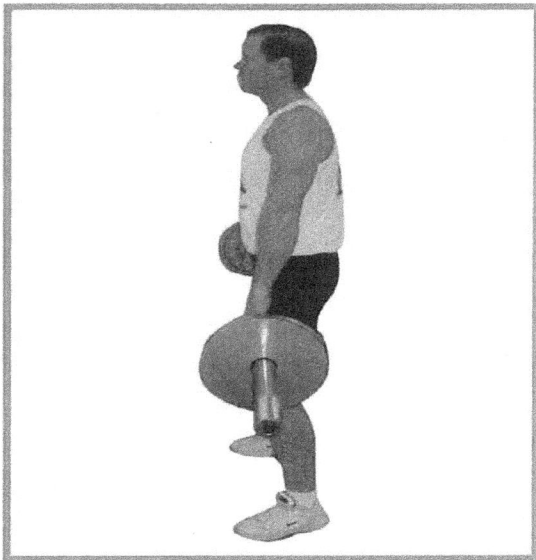

Start

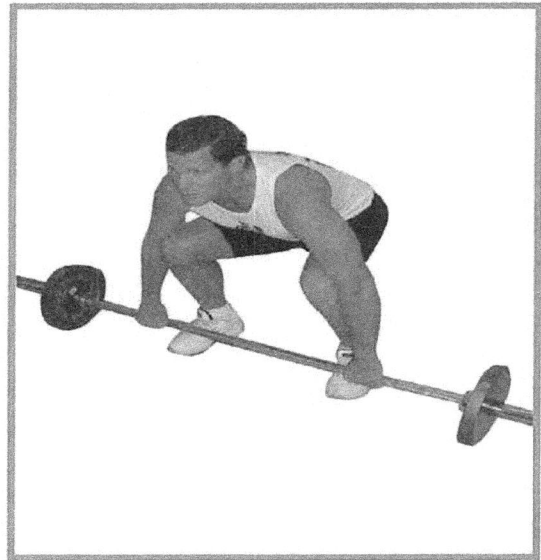

Finish

* Start with feet slightly wider than your shoulders, toes pointed out slightly.
* Grab bar just outside of your knees, look forward, keep you back flat.
* Stand up to straight position.
* Come back down to start position.

Mike's Special Pointer:
Concentrate on form when doing exercise. Keep flat footed and don't let your knees go forward of your toes.

Dumbbell Rows: One Arm

Target Area – Latissimus (middle and outer back)

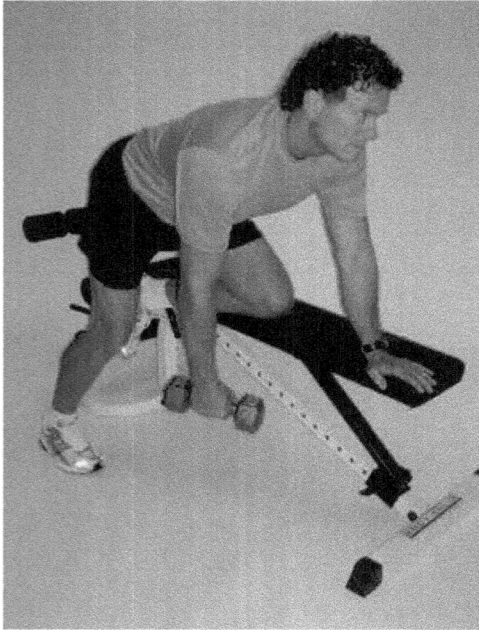

Start

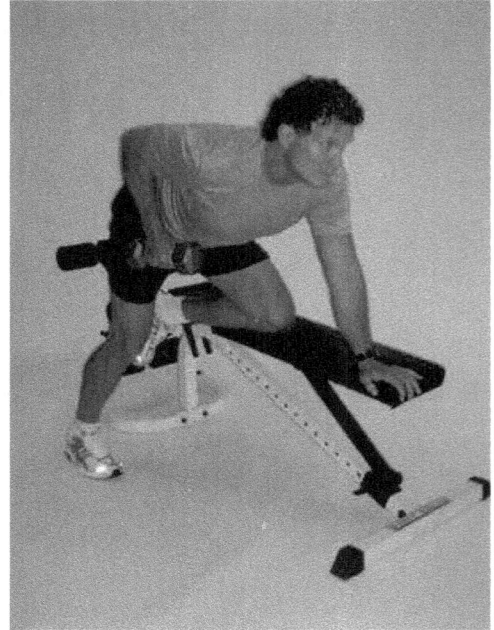

Finish

- On a flat bench, put your knee up for support, (the knee of the leg opposite of the hand that will be doing the exercise).
- Place your other hand down for support.
- Allow the dumbbell to hang in a full stretch.
- Pull the weight up and slightly back so that your hand ends up at your rib cage in the up position.
- Lower the weight to a stretch position, allow your shoulder to drop down slightly for a better stretch.

Mike's Special Pointer:

When you pull up, your forearm should stay approximately straight up and down throughout the exercise. A common mistake is to pull the wrist up under the body so that the forearm angles forward.

Bicep Curls - Bar - Regular Grip

<u>TARGET AREA -</u>   <u>Biceps - front of upper arms</u>

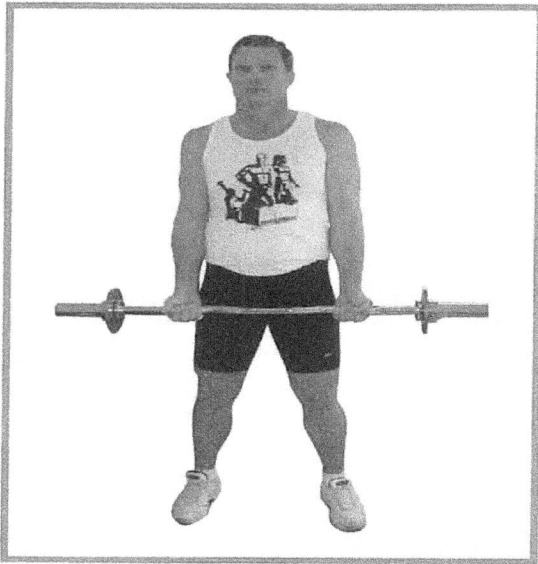

Start

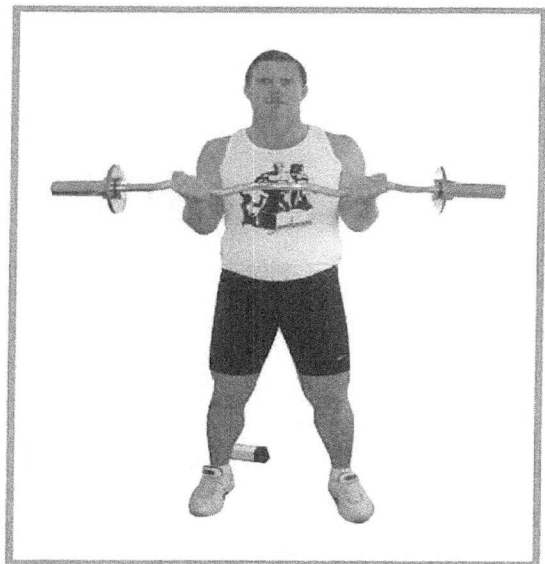

Finish

* Grab bar a little wider than shoulder width- special curl bar should allow palms to turn in slightly, feet about shoulder's width apart, soft knees.
* Keeping elbows down, curl the bar up towards the top of chest.
* Lower it back to start position.

Mike's Special Pointer:
Perhaps the most common mistake on bar curls is to bring the elbows forward at the top of the movement. This takes a lot of stress off the bicep muscle and puts it in the joint- exactly what you don't want when you do curls.

Leg Curls - Kneeling

TARGET AREA -   **Hamstrings - back of upper legs**

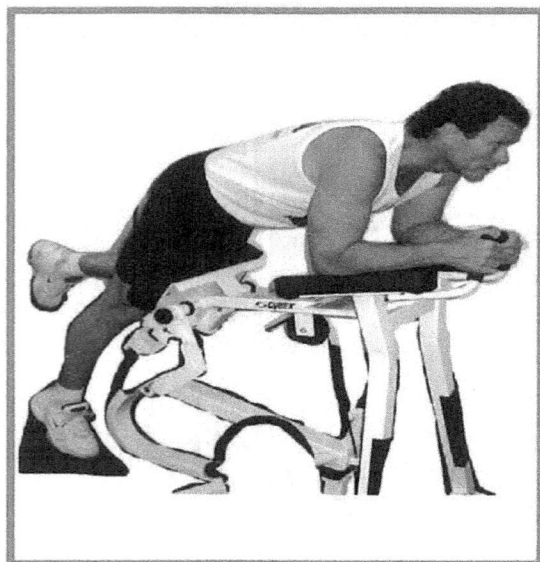

Start

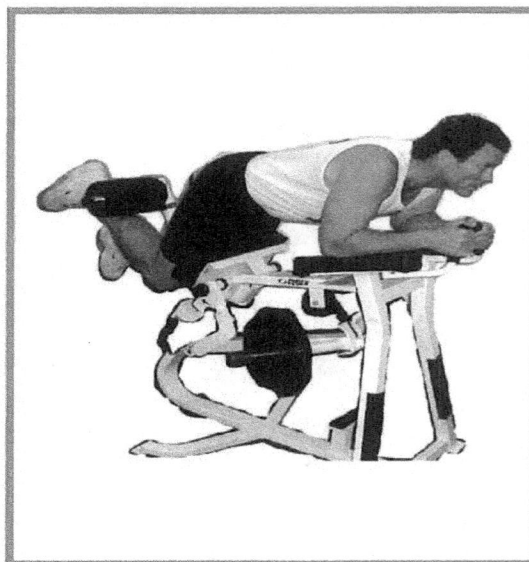

Finish

* Position machine so that you are kneeling on one pad, working ankle behind the lower pad, and upper body resting on forearm pads.
* Look ahead, pull your lower leg up as high as you can, to at least a 90 degree bend of the knee.
* Lower the weight back down until your leg is straight, but be careful not to let the pad go too far, hyper-extending your knee.

Mike's Special Pointer:
This is one of the best hamstring exercises there is, but it's not done very often. It's good for athletes that run in their sport because the exercise more closely mimics the running movement.

Smith Machine - Calf Raises

__TARGET AREA -__   __Calves - back of lower legs__

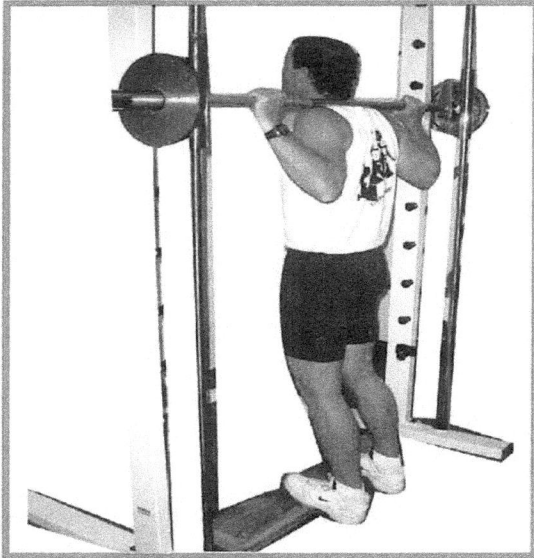

Start

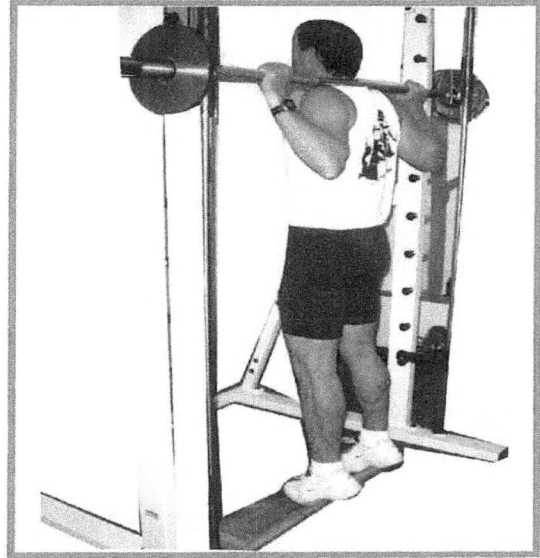

Finish

* Place bar a little higher than shoulder's width, put on the floor a piece of 2"x 4" or anything that allows your heels to fall off the edge, and set the back edge approximately under the bar.
* Get under the bar, place it across your very upper back, not on the base of your neck, grab bar wherever it's comfortable, step up on the step so the balls of your feet are squarely on the surface with your heels and arch over the edge.
* Unlatch the bar. Go down into a full stretch.
* Push up on your toes as high as possible without locking your knees.
* Come back down to the start position.

Mike's Special Pointer:
Try to get a full range of motion when doing calf exercises. Drop those heels as low as possible- feel the stretch. Come back up so that your heels go higher than your toes.

Pull Downs: Front

Target Area – Latissimus (middle and outer back)

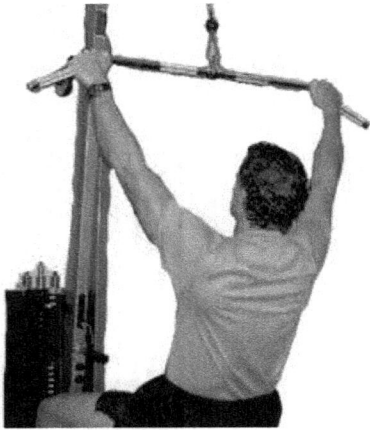
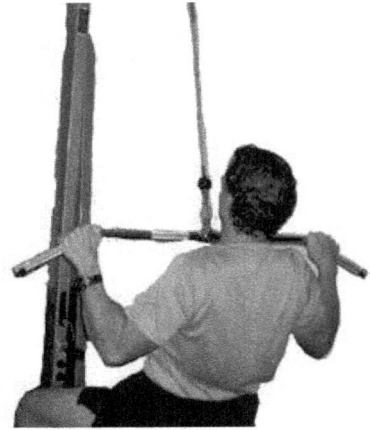

Start   **Finish**

- Position hands wider than your shoulders, palms facing out forward, away from you.
- Pull straight down until the bar comes at or below your chin.
- Raise the bar back up to the starting position, be sure your arms are fully extended giving you a full stretch.

Mike's Special Pointer:

When coming down, don't turn your forearms down so that your palms angle down. When in the finish position, your palms should be facing straight ahead.

Leg Extensions

Target Area – Quadriceps (front of upper legs)

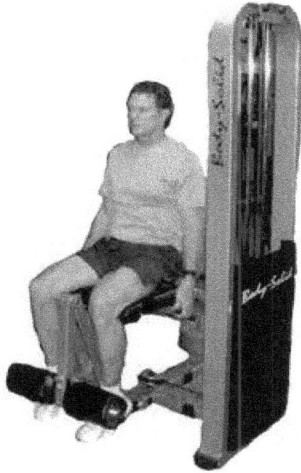 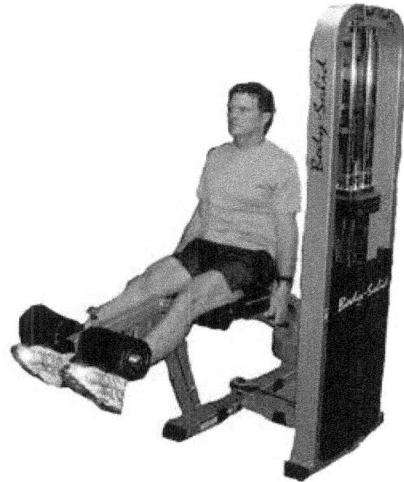

Start   **Finish**

- Sit with your back flat against the pad, hook your feet behind the pads.
- Extend your feet so they go up towards the ceiling – your feet should be relaxed.
- Pause at the top with your legs fully extended.
- Slowly lower your legs back down to the starting position.

Mike's Special Pointer:

Come all the way up and pause at the top. Be sure to lower the weight back down as opposed to just letting gravity do it.

Concentration Curls

TARGET AREA -   Biceps - front of upper arms

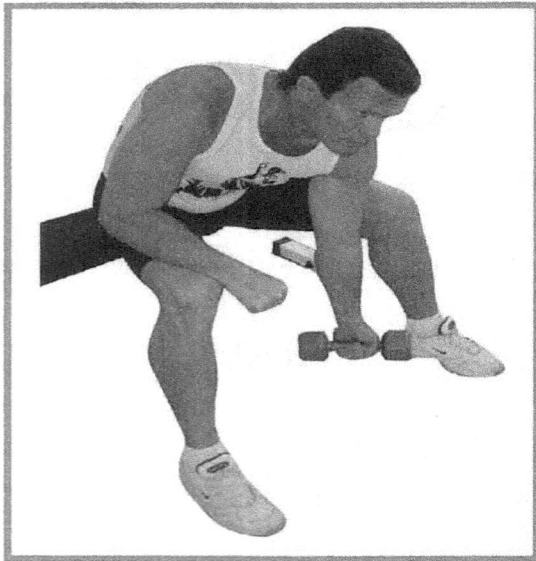

Start

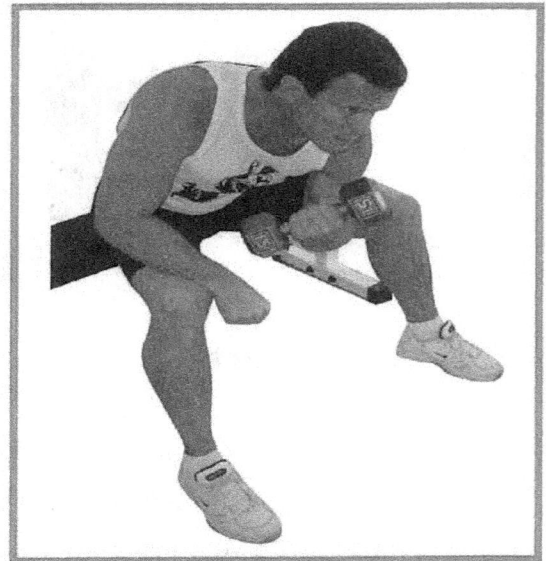

Finish

*   Sit sideways on a bench or chair and spread your legs.
*   Put non-working arm so that it supports upper body weight just above the knee.
*   Hang the working arm down, palm facing towards your other leg, back of upper arm braced against the inside of your leg near your knee.
*   Curl the weight up, keeping your upper body steady- go as high as you can.
*   Lower the weight back down to start position.

Mike's Special Pointer:
Come all the way down until your arm is straight. Doing bicep curls with a short range of motion can shorten your tendons and make you more prone to injury.

Calf Raise: Reverse, Machine

Target Area – Anterior Tibialis (front of lower leg)

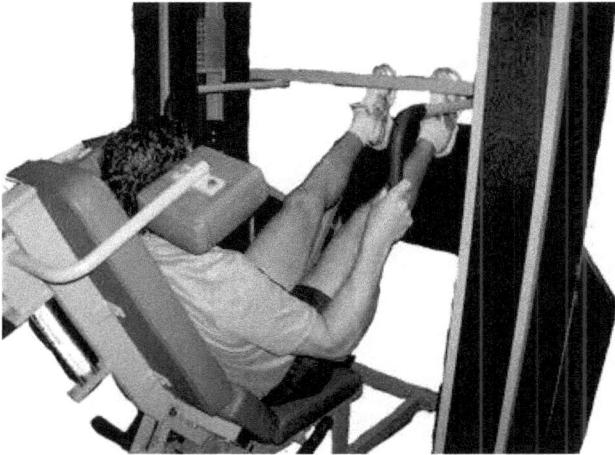 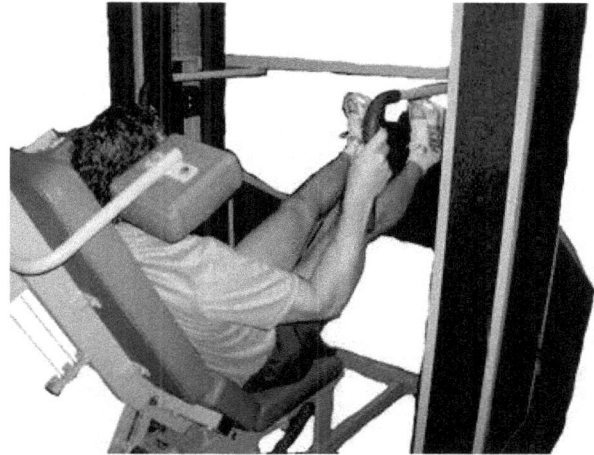

Start   **Finish**

- Set your seat so that you can sit with your knees slightly bent with the toes of your feet over the top of the foot pad.
- Point your toes to stretch the fronts of your lower legs.
- While being careful to keep the exact same angle of your knees, push with your heels as you pull your toes back towards you, the weight stack will move only slightly.
- Go back to the stretch position

Mike's Special Pointer:

This is a great exercise for helping to cure shin splints. If you've had these problems in the past, do this exercise faithfully 2-3 times per week for the best results.

Inner Thigh Machine

TARGET AREA -   Inner Thighs

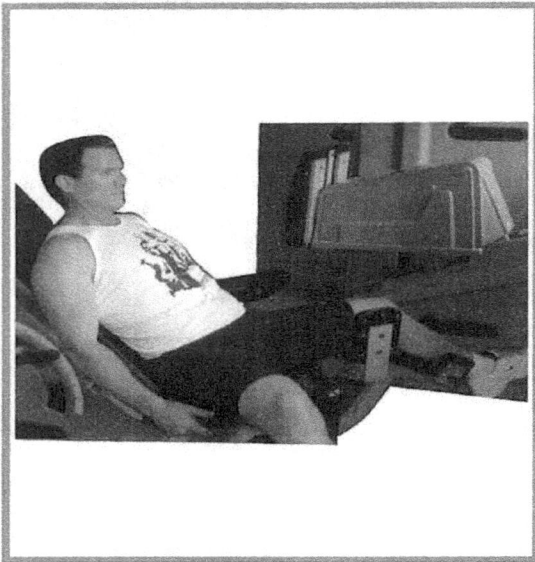

Start

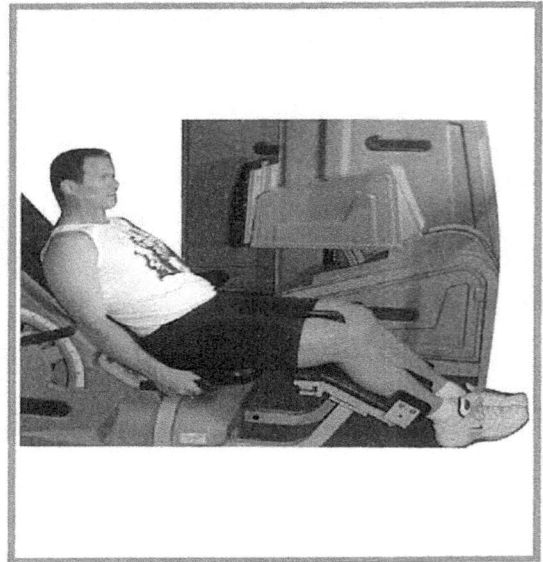

Finish

* Set machine so that you can get a full stretch without the weight touching down in the start position. Sit back in seat, position pads inside the legs.
* Hold onto handles.
* Allow machine to stretch your inner thighs as knees spread further apart.
* Squeeze your legs back together until pads meet in front of you.
* Ease your legs back apart to full stretch.

Mike's Special Pointer:
When doing this exercise, think of pushing with your knees, not your feet. Also, it's important to keep your legs straight up. Don't turn your heels in when pulling together.

Outer Thigh Machine

TARGET AREA -   Outer Thighs

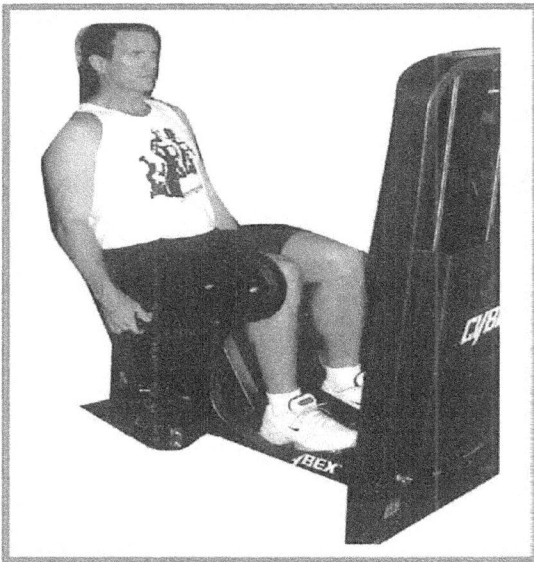

Start

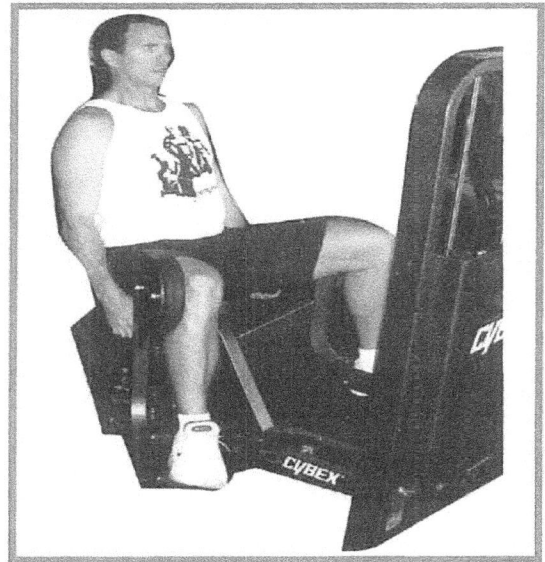

Finish

* Sit in seat, knee pads should be on the outside of your legs.
* Hold hand grips.
* Push out as far as you can, pause, and come back out to start position.

Mike's Special Pointer:
You'll get a lot more out of this exercise if you hold the weight out
in the finish position for at least 1 second. Go out as far as you can,
hold it there, then return slowly.

Dumbbell Low Back lifts

TARGET AREA -   Lower Back

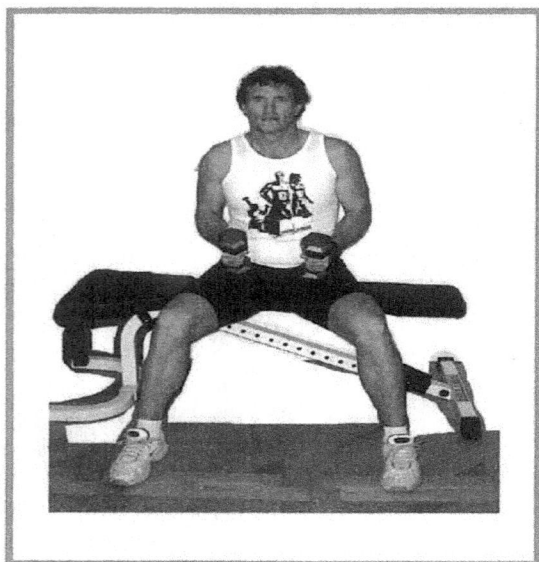

Start

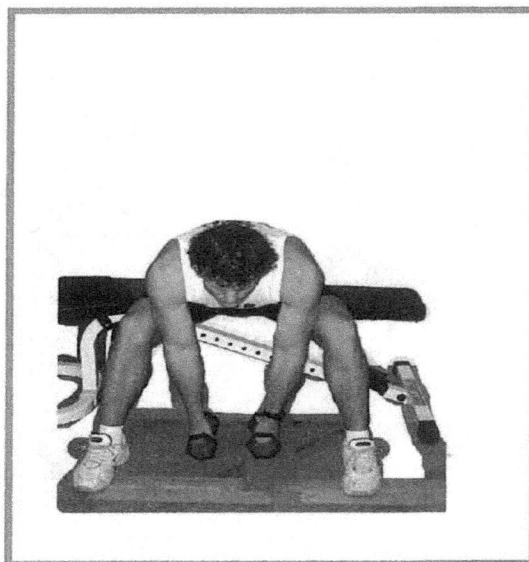

Finish

* Sit on a chair or on a bench, feet spread apart about shoulder's width, dumbbells held above your lap
* Bend down at the waist, lowering the dumbbells to where they almost touch the floor.
* Come back up until you are sitting up straight, holding the dumbbells just above your thighs.

Mike's Special Pointer:
Try & keep your back flat instead of rounded as you go up and down to isolate the low back muscles. Keep the weights light at first until you have mastered the form.

Pain Free Functional Strength Workout – Advanced Male: Chest, Shoulders, Triceps, Abs, Traps

Quick Sheet – Review and Additional Instructions

Before Starting:

* Be sure you have a way to make small increases when using weights or dumbbells less than 50 pounds.

* Take one workout to get your starting weight established for each exercise. For all exercises, find the weight that you can get one set of 10 reps moderately easy.

* Write down all these starting weights on your *Pain Free Functional Strength* workout chart, just above the word "weight".

* Each exercise is explained in detail in the pages that follow your workout chart.

Pain Free Functional Strength: The Workout

* Your first workout – Do 3 sets of 8 reps for each exercise. (Except for the calf raises, abdominal exercises, shoulder shrugs and wrist curls. Instead of doing 8, 9, 10, 11 and 12 reps you will use 11, 12, 13, 14, and 15 reps for these exercises instead)

* Workout Number 2 – do 3 sets of 9 reps

* Workout Number 3 – do 3 sets of 10 reps

* Workout Number 4 – do 3 sets of 11 reps

* Workout Number 5 – do 3 sets of 12 reps

* Workout Number 6 – Increase the weight by only 5 to 10 percent for each exercise. But now drop your reps back to 3 sets of 8

* Workout Number 7 – do 3 sets of 9 reps

* Workout Number 8 – do 3 sets of 10 reps

* Workout Number 9 – do 3 sets of 11 reps

* Workout Number 10 – do 3 sets of 12 reps

* Workout Number 11 - Increase the weights by 5 to 10 percent once again on those exercises that you got 3 sets of 12 on during the last workout. Continue the normal progression on all the other exercises, or use the next 5 workouts to "even it out" (as described in chapter 6)

* Continue as long as you can using this pattern

* *Pain Free Functional Strength* ends on an exercise when you can no longer get the number of reps that the workout calls for 2 workouts in a row.

* For the remaining workouts, continue doing those exercises that came to an end for at least your 3 sets of 8 reps, while working the progression for the remaining exercises. When all the exercises

have come to their anticipated end, you have finished *Pain Free Functional Strength* – Congratulations!

What now? Pick all new exercises and start back at the beginning. Or continue on this workout but decrease the weight by 25%-33% and do 5, 6, and 7 reps instead of 8 through 12.

Additional exercises and instructions.

1.   Dumbbell Side Raises- Do 1 to 2 sets of 12 reps, gradually building up to a total of 25 reps.
2.   Bicycle Sit Ups - Do 1 to 2 sets of 15 reps, build up to 30 or more reps.

Workout Chart - For 8, 9, 10, 11 and 12 reps – Advanced Male: Chest, Shoulders, Triceps, Abs, Traps

(Cross off rep counts as you progress through workouts)

Exercise #1: Dumbbell Bench Press	Weight:	8,9,10,11,12		8,9,10,11,12		8,9,10,11,12
		8,9,10,11,12		8,9,10,11,12		8,9,10,11,12
		8,9,10,11,12		8,9,10,11,12		8,9,10,11,12
Exercise #2: Dumbbell Triceps Ext. (on back)	Weight:	8,9,10,11,12		8,9,10,11,12		8,9,10,11,12
		8,9,10,11,12		8,9,10,11,12		8,9,10,11,12
		8,9,10,11,12		8,9,10,11,12		8,9,10,11,12
Exercise #3: Dumbbell Military Press Standing, Twist	Weight:	8,9,10,11,12		8,9,10,11,12		8,9,10,11,12
		8,9,10,11,12		8,9,10,11,12		8,9,10,11,12
		8,9,10,11,12		8,9,10,11,12		8,9,10,11,12
Exercise #4: Shrugs, Bar (10,11,12,13,14 reps)	Weight:	10,11,12,13,14		10,11,12,13,14		10,11,12,13,14
		10,11,12,13,14		10,11,12,13,14		10,11,12,13,14
		10,11,12,13,14		10,11,12,13,14		10,11,12,13,14
Exercise #5: Dumbbell Lateral Raise, Seated, Bent Over (Do 2 sets only)	Weight:	8,9,10,11,12		8,9,10,11,12		8,9,10,11,12
		8,9,10,11,12		8,9,10,11,12		8,9,10,11,12
		8,9,10,11,12		8,9,10,11,12		8,9,10,11,12
Exercise #6: Chest Flies, Cable	Weight:	8,9,10,11,12		8,9,10,11,12		8,9,10,11,12
		8,9,10,11,12		8,9,10,11,12		8,9,10,11,12
		8,9,10,11,12		8,9,10,11,12		8,9,10,11,12
Exercise #7: Bench Press Close Grip	Weight:	8,9,10,11,12		8,9,10,11,12		8,9,10,11,12
		8,9,10,11,12		8,9,10,11,12		8,9,10,11,12
		8,9,10,11,12		8,9,10,11,12		8,9,10,11,12
Exercise #8: Upright Rows	Weight:	8,9,10,11,12		8,9,10,11,12		8,9,10,11,12
		8,9,10,11,12		8,9,10,11,12		8,9,10,11,12
		8,9,10,11,12		8,9,10,11,12		8,9,10,11,12
Exercise #9: Dips, Assisted	Weight:	8,9,10,11,12		8,9,10,11,12		8,9,10,11,12
		8,9,10,11,12		8,9,10,11,12		8,9,10,11,12
		8,9,10,11,12		8,9,10,11,12		8,9,10,11,12

Additional exercises and instructions.

1. Dumbbell Side Raises- Do 1 to 2 sets of 12 reps, gradually building up to a total of 25 reps.
2. Bicycle Sit Ups - Do 1 to 2 sets of 15 reps, build up to 30 or more reps.

Dumbbell Bench Press

Target Area – Pectorals (chest)

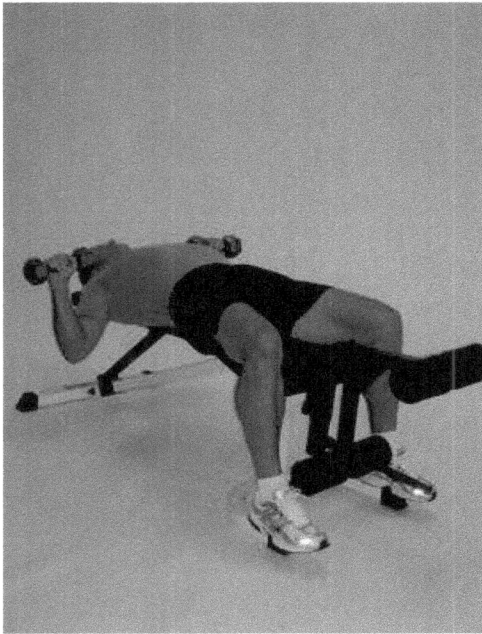

Start

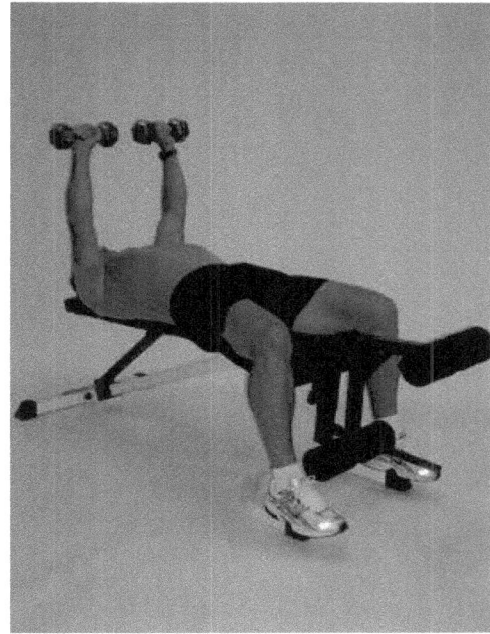

Finish

- Lay flat on your back, putting your feet up is optional.
- Start with the weights wider than your shoulders, elbows at or slightly below the bench.
- Push up and allow the weights to come close together at the top without touching.
- Don't lock out your elbows.
- Come back down to the start position, but don't let your forearms angle out – keep them straight up.

Mike's Special Pointer:

When pushing up, it's OK if your elbows are slightly forward. Many people can develop shoulder injuries if they try and force their elbows way back while doing the exercise.

Dumbbell Triceps Extension: On Back

Target Area – Triceps (back of upper arms)

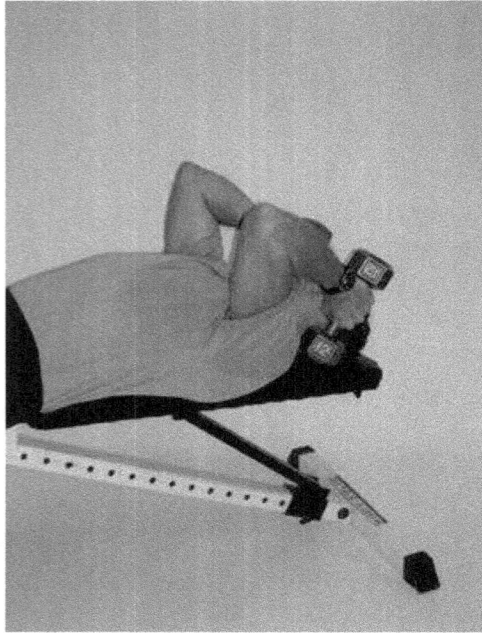

Start

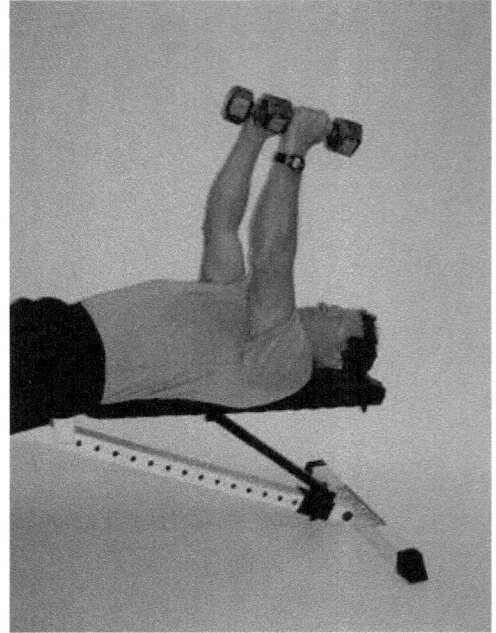

Finish

- Lay flat on a bench, knees up or down according to your preference, dumbbells held straight up, palms facing towards each other.
- Keeping elbows in and up, lower the weights so your hands come approximately to your ears.
- Push back up to the start position.

Mike's Special Pointer:

Keep those elbows in the same place. They tend to want to move backwards and forwards as you do the movements. Don't let that happen though – keep them stationary.

Dumbbell Military Press (Standing) - Twisting

TARGET AREA -   Deltoids - shoulders

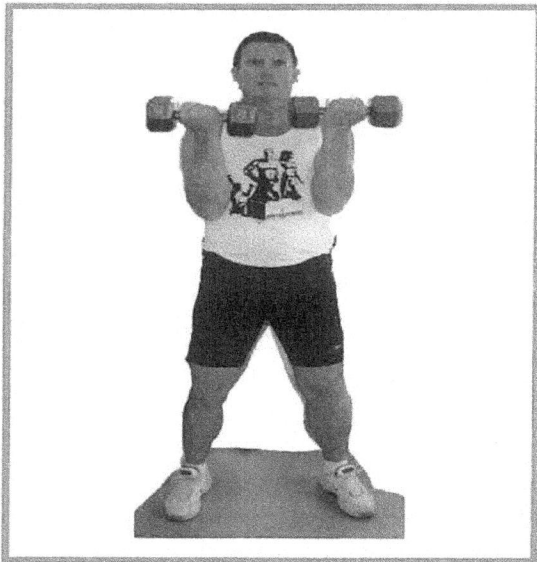

Start

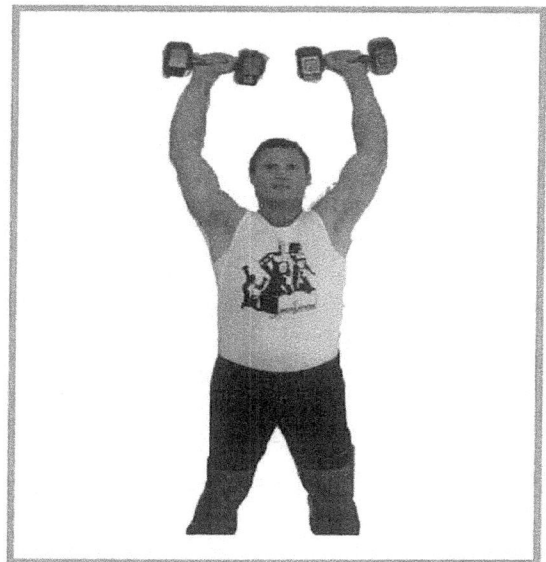

Finish

* This exercise can be done either sitting or standing (as illustrated above).
* Hold the weights so palms face you, hands just below chin level.
* Push up and as you do rotate the dumbbells so that the palms turn towards each other and then finally end up palms facing forward once you have arrived at the top.
* Your knees should be slightly bent but not locked
* Come back to the start position, rotate the opposite way as on the way up.

Mike's Special Pointer:
Be careful not to hit yourself with the dumbbells as you rotate your arms.
Check in the mirror to make sure you are well in the clear.

Shrugs - Bar

TARGET AREA -   **Trapezius - upper back**

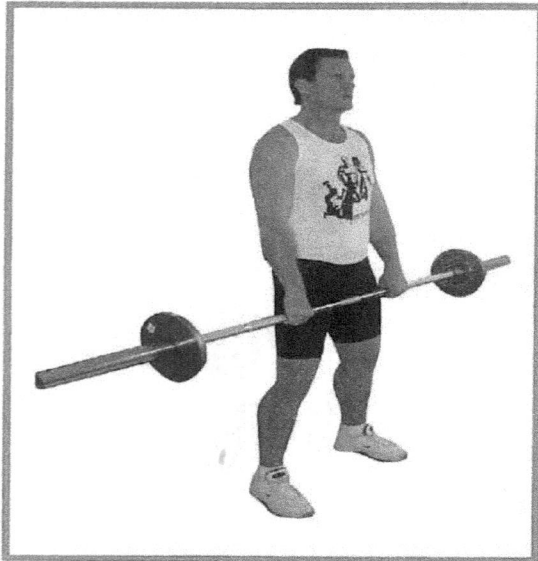

Start

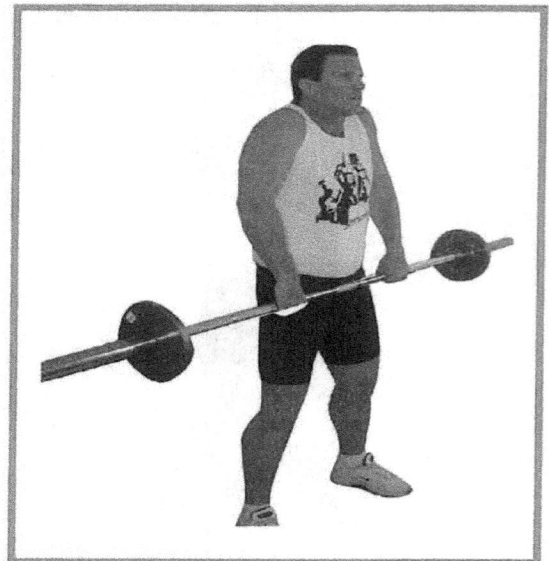

Finish

* Place your feet wider than your shoulders, grab bar at about shoulder's width, palms facing you, keep a soft bend in your knees.
* Shrug your shoulders up as high as you can without hardly any bend in your elbows.
* Come back down and allow the bar to stretch all the way down.

Mike's Special Pointer:
Try pausing at the top for a full count of 2-3 seconds. Shrugs are such a short range movement that this pause seems to really help work the muscles.

Dumbbell Lateral Raise - Bent Over - Seated

TARGET AREA -   Deltoids - back of shoulders

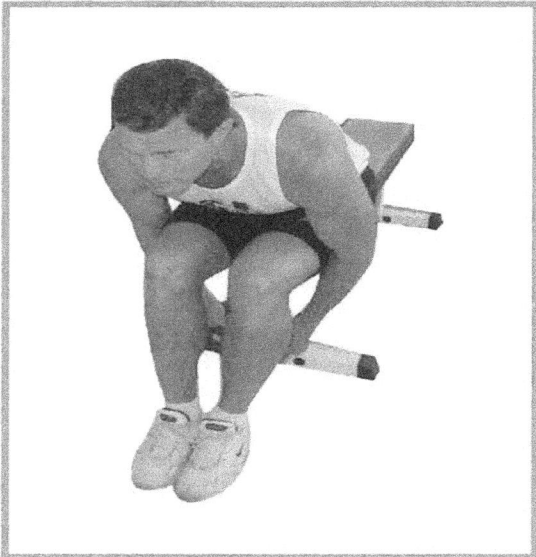

Start

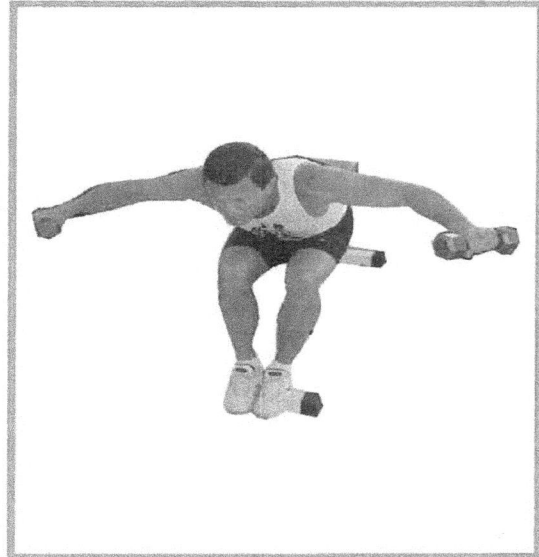

Finish

* Sit on the edge of a bench or on a chair, bend over and hold weights under legs, chin up, back flat.
* Extend your arms out and come up to where forearms are pointed to the sides, but slightly forward.
* Lower back down to start position under legs.

Mike's Special Pointer:
Stay down while doing this exercise. The tendency is to sit more upright, changing the target area of the exercise.

Chest Flies: Cable

Target Area – Pectorals (chest)

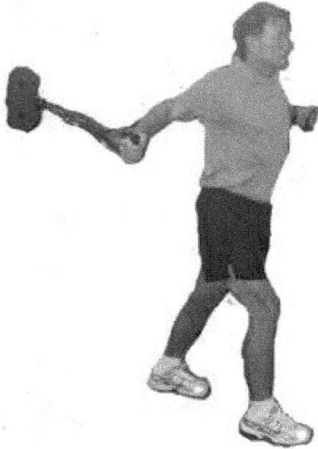

Start

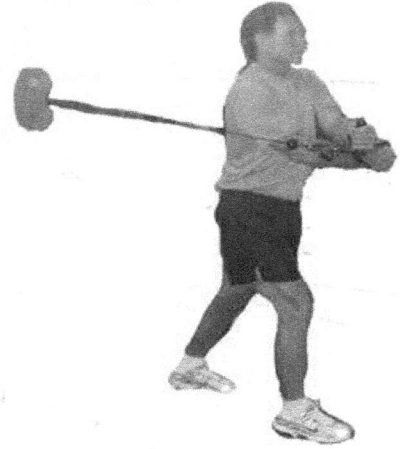

Finish

- Put handles on upper part of cable machine.
- Grab one handle, move over sideways far enough to grab other handle, come back to center, feet nearly together, knees bent slightly, arms extended up and out.
- With palms forward in start position, pull handles in front of you until they cross, keep elbows bent slightly the whole time.
- Come back up to a stretch.

Mike's Special Pointer:

I like to cross my hands differently after each repetition, right over left, left over right, etc. This ensures equal use of the muscles.

Bench Press - Close Grip

TARGET AREA -   Pectorals & Triceps - chest and back of upper arms

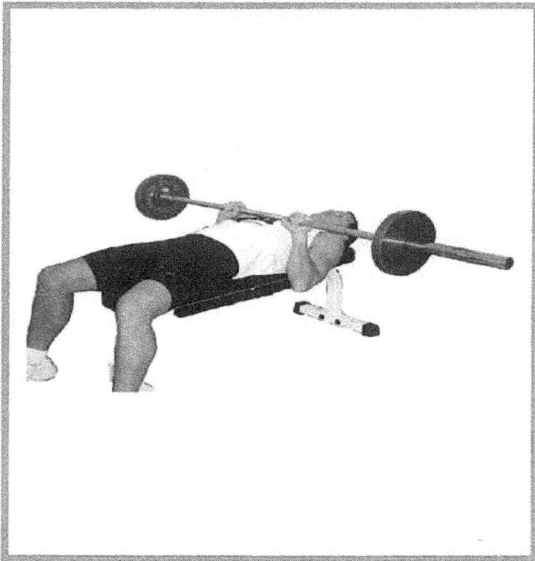

Start

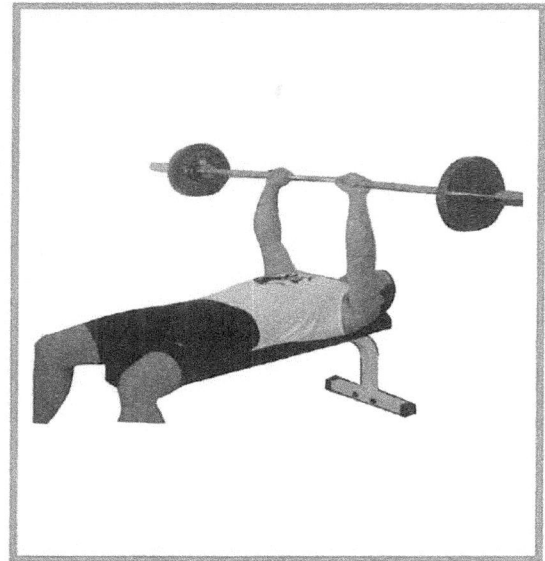

Finish

* Lay flat on bench, grab bar a little narrower than your shoulders.
* Thumbs can be on either side of the bar as a matter of personal preference.
* With the bar at or slightly below your sternum (the bone at the center of your chest), push up.
* Allow the bar to come forward so that when your arms are straight (but not locked) the bar is about over your chin.
* Lower the bar to the starting position.

Mike's Special Pointer:
Keep your elbows in (tight up against your sides) when you do this exercise. You should really feel it in the tricep muscles when you do it.

Dumbbell Upright Rows

Target Area – Deltoids (shoulders)

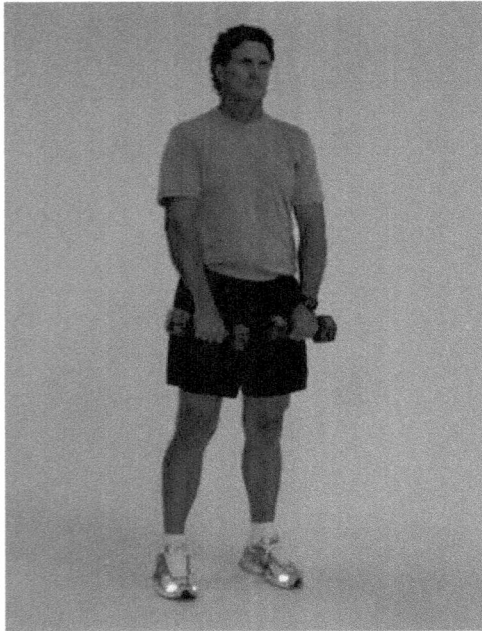

Start

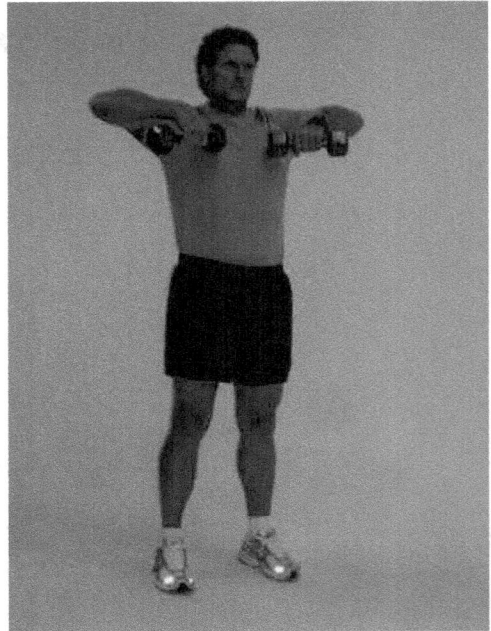

Finish

- Let the weights hang in front of you, palms facing towards you.
- Bring the weights up in a straight line, until your hands almost reach your arm pits.
- Lower the weights back down to the starting position.

Mike's Special Pointer:

Keep your posture straight. Don't lean back as you raise the weights up.

Dips - Assisted

TARGET AREA -   Pectorals & Triceps - chest and back of upper arms

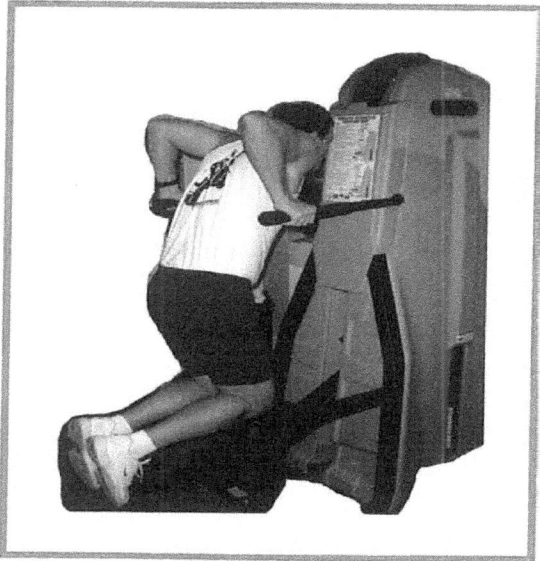

Start

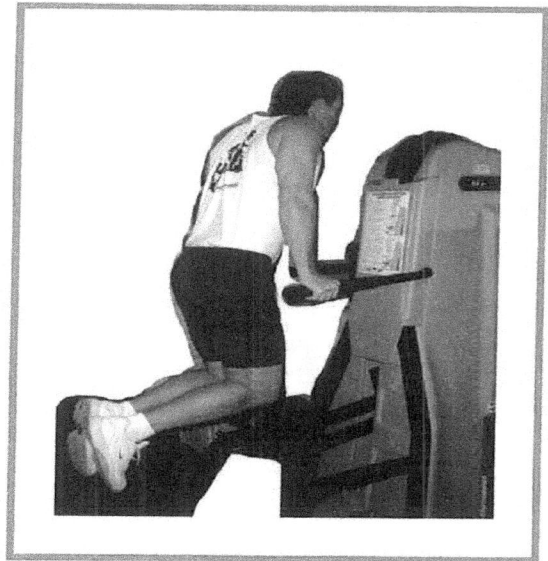

Finish

* Set weight with the weight stack pin, the more weight you use the easier the exercise.
* Grab bars at your sides with palms facing in, step or kneel onto the assisting pad, extend your arms fully without locking your elbows.
* Keeping elbows back, come down into a stretch.
* Push back up to start position.

Mike's Special Pointer:
To work your triceps harder, keep your elbows back when coming down and pushing up. It's OK to lean slightly forward.

Dumbbell Side Raises

TARGET AREA - Obliques - sides of abdominials

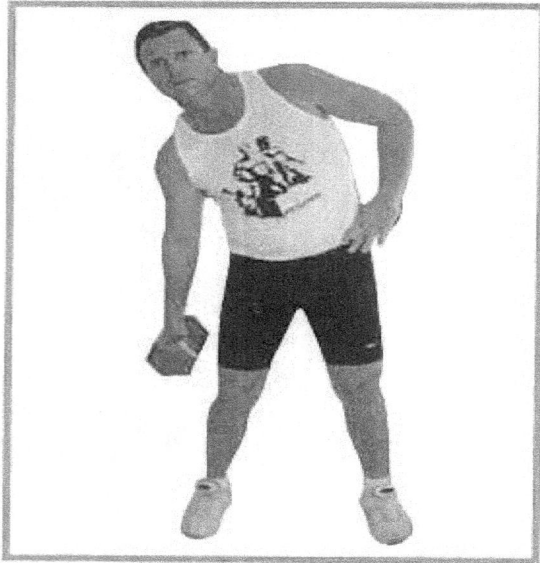

Start

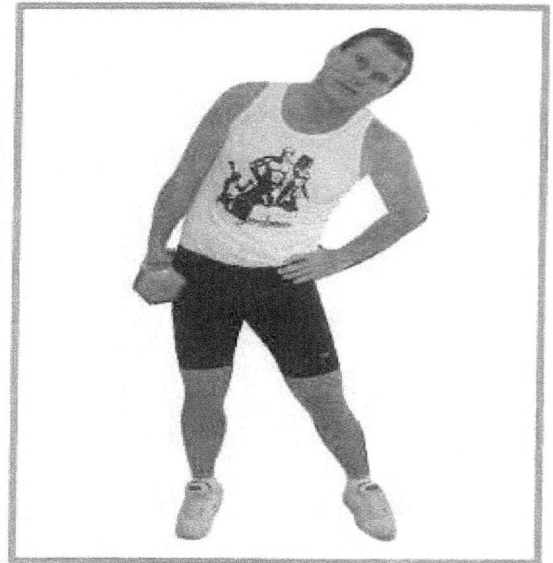

Finish

* Grab a dumbbell, stand with feet about shoulder's width apart, put non-working hand on hip.
* Lower weight sideways to a point just above the knee.
* Raise the weight the other way as high as you can keeping your hips square.

Mike's Special Pointer:
Be sure to go over sideways. The tendency is to turn slightly forward, decreasing the effectiveness of the exercise.

Sit Ups - Bicycle

TARGET AREA -   Abdominals & Obliques - front & sides of torso

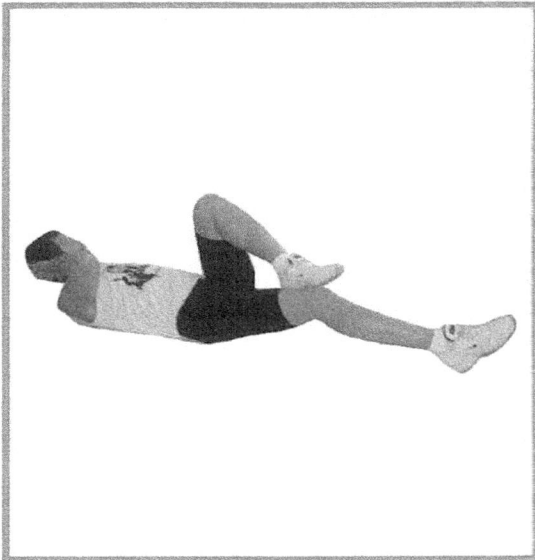

Start

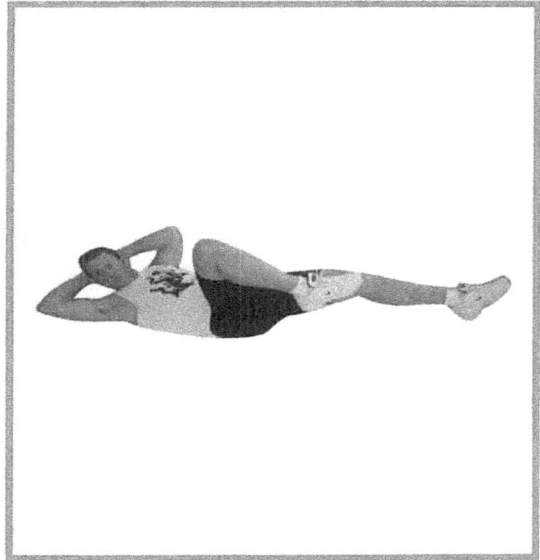

Finish

* Lay flat on your back on the floor or a mat, lightly clasp your fingers behind your head, raise both feet off the floor with knees slightly bent.
* Bring one knee up as the opposite elbow turns toward it.
* Stop well short of the elbow touching the knee.
* Next, bring the other leg in as the original leg extends out.
* While this is happening you're pivoting your upper body the other way so that your other elbow is moving towards your opposite knee.
* Keep crisscrossing until you've done the desired number of repetitions.

Mike's Special Pointer:
Don't swing your shoulders side to side on the floor. Think of a pivot rod attached to the top of your head, not allowing your head to move all around- only pivot. That's the action you're looking for.

Advanced Female:

Pain Free Functional Strength Workout – Advanced Female: Legs, Upper and Lower Back, Biceps

Quick Sheet – Review and Additional Instructions

Before Starting:

* Be sure you have a way to make small increases when using weights or dumbbells less than 50 pounds.

* Take one workout to get your starting weight established for each exercise. For all exercises, find the weight that you can get one set of 10 reps moderately easy.

* Write down all these starting weights on your *Pain Free Functional Strength* workout chart, just above the word "weight".

* Each exercise is explained in detail in the pages that follow your workout chart.

Pain Free Functional Strength: The Workout

* Your first workout – Do 3 sets of 8 reps for each exercise. (Except for the calf raises, abdominal exercises, shoulder shrugs and wrist curls. Instead of doing 8, 9, 10, 11 and 12 reps you will use 11, 12, 13, 14, and 15 reps for these exercises instead)

* Workout Number 2 – do 3 sets of 9 reps

* Workout Number 3 – do 3 sets of 10 reps

* Workout Number 4 – do 3 sets of 11 reps

* Workout Number 5 – do 3 sets of 12 reps

* Workout Number 6 – Increase the weight by only 5 to 10 percent for each exercise. But now drop your reps back to 3 sets of 8

* Workout Number 7 – do 3 sets of 9 reps

* Workout Number 8 – do 3 sets of 10 reps

* Workout Number 9 – do 3 sets of 11 reps

* Workout Number 10 – do 3 sets of 12 reps

* Workout Number 11 - Increase the weights by 5 to 10 percent once again on those exercises that you got 3 sets of 12 on during the last workout. Continue the normal progression on all the other exercises, or use the next 5 workouts to "even it out" (as described in chapter 6)

* Continue as long as you can using this pattern

* *Pain Free Functional Strength* ends on an exercise when you can no longer get the number of reps that the workout calls for 2 workouts in a row.

* For the remaining workouts, continue doing those exercises that came to an end for at least your 3 sets of 8 reps, while working the progression for the remaining exercises. When all the exercises have come to their anticipated end, you have finished *Pain Free Functional Strength* – Congratulations!

What now? Pick all new exercises and start back at the beginning. Or continue on this workout but decrease the weight by 25-33% and do 5, 6, and 7 reps instead of 8 through 12.

Additional Instructions:

This is one of 2 workouts for the advanced female. Do this work out 2 or 3 days per week, alternating it with the other. Your week will look something like this: Monday and Thursday the legs, lats and biceps workout, Tuesday and Friday the chest, shoulders and abs workout. Rest Saturday and Sunday. Or you could also do the first workout on Monday, Wednesday and Friday and the second Tuesday, Thursday and Saturday, rest Sunday.

Workout Chart - For 8, 9, 10, 11 and 12 reps – Advanced Female: Legs, Upper Back, Biceps, Lower Back

(Cross off rep counts as you progress through workouts)

Exercise	Weight	Set 1	Set 2	Set 3
Exercise #1: Leg Extensions	Weight: _____ _____ _____	8,9,10,11,12 8,9,10,11,12 8,9,10,11,12	8,9,10,11,12 8,9,10,11,12 8,9,10,11,12	8,9,10,11,12 8,9,10,11,12 8,9,10,11,12
Exercise #2: Dumbbell Pullovers	Weight: _____ _____ _____	8,9,10,11,12 8,9,10,11,12 8,9,10,11,12	8,9,10,11,12 8,9,10,11,12 8,9,10,11,12	8,9,10,11,12 8,9,10,11,12 8,9,10,11,12
Exercise #3: Calf Raises, Machine, Standing	Weight: _____ _____ _____	8,9,10,11,12 8,9,10,11,12 8,9,10,11,12	8,9,10,11,12 8,9,10,11,12 8,9,10,11,12	8,9,10,11,12 8,9,10,11,12 8,9,10,11,12
Exercise #4: Bar Biceps Curls Close Grip	Weight: _____ _____ _____	8,9,10,11,12 8,9,10,11,12 8,9,10,11,12	8,9,10,11,12 8,9,10,11,12 8,9,10,11,12	8,9,10,11,12 8,9,10,11,12 8,9,10,11,12
Exercise #5: Rows, Low Cable, Narrow Grip	Weight: _____ _____ _____	8,9,10,11,12 8,9,10,11,12 8,9,10,11,12	8,9,10,11,12 8,9,10,11,12 8,9,10,11,12	8,9,10,11,12 8,9,10,11,12 8,9,10,11,12
Exercise #6: Lunges, Stationary	Weight: _____ _____ _____	8,9,10,11,12 8,9,10,11,12 8,9,10,11,12	8,9,10,11,12 8,9,10,11,12 8,9,10,11,12	8,9,10,11,12 8,9,10,11,12 8,9,10,11,12
Exercise #7: Dumbbell Dead Lifts	Weight: _____ _____ _____	8,9,10,11,12 8,9,10,11,12 8,9,10,11,12	8,9,10,11,12 8,9,10,11,12 8,9,10,11,12	8,9,10,11,12 8,9,10,11,12 8,9,10,11,12
Exercise #8: Leg Curls, Lying On Stomach	Weight: _____ _____ _____	8,9,10,11,12 8,9,10,11,12 8,9,10,11,12	8,9,10,11,12 8,9,10,11,12 8,9,10,11,12	8,9,10,11,12 8,9,10,11,12 8,9,10,11,12
Exercise #9: Inner Thigh Machine (Do 2 sets)	Weight: _____ _____ _____	8,9,10,11,12 8,9,10,11,12 8,9,10,11,12	8,9,10,11,12 8,9,10,11,12 8,9,10,11,12	8,9,10,11,12 8,9,10,11,12 8,9,10,11,12

Exercise #10: outer Thigh Machine (Do 2 sets)	**Weight:**	8,9,10,11,12		8,9,10,11,12		8,9,10,11,12
		8,9,10,11,12		8,9,10,11,12		8,9,10,11,12
		8,9,10,11,12		8,9,10,11,12		8,9,10,11,12
Exercise #11: Concentration Curls	**Weight:**	8,9,10,11,12		8,9,10,11,12		8,9,10,11,12
		8,9,10,11,12		8,9,10,11,12		8,9,10,11,12
		8,9,10,11,12		8,9,10,11,12		8,9,10,11,12
Exercise #12: Lower Back Machine	**Weight:**	8,9,10,11,12		8,9,10,11,12		8,9,10,11,12
		8,9,10,11,12		8,9,10,11,12		8,9,10,11,12
		8,9,10,11,12		8,9,10,11,12		8,9,10,11,12

Leg Extensions

Target Area – Quadriceps (front of upper legs)

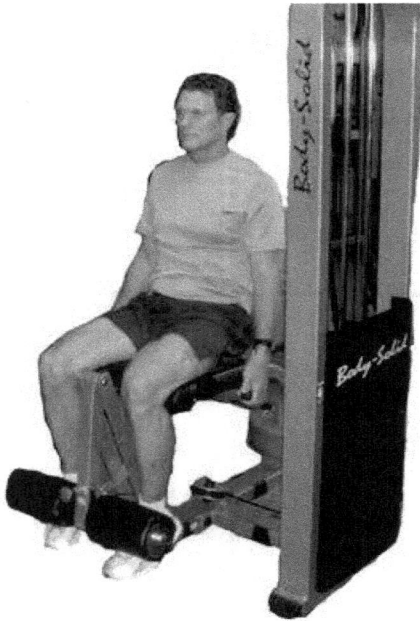

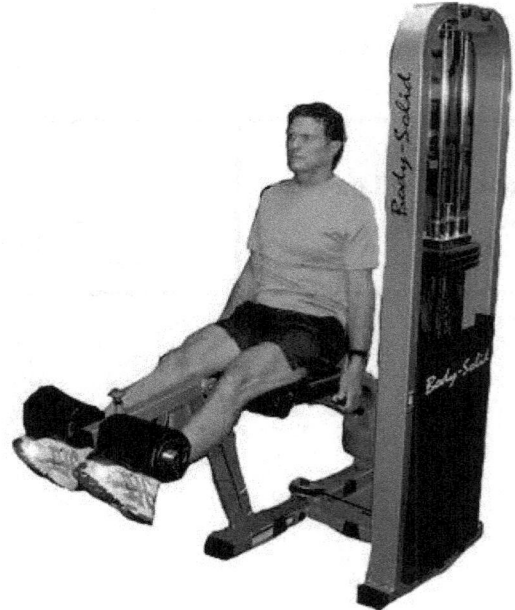

Start   **Finish**

- Sit with your back flat against the pad, hook your feet behind the pads.
- Extend your feet so they go up towards the ceiling – your feet should be relaxed.
- Pause at the top with your legs fully extended.
- Slowly lower your legs back down to the starting position.

Mike's Special Pointer:

Come all the way up and pause at the top. Be sure to lower the weight back down as opposed to just letting gravity do it.

Dumbbell Pullovers

Target Area – Latissimus (middle and outer back)

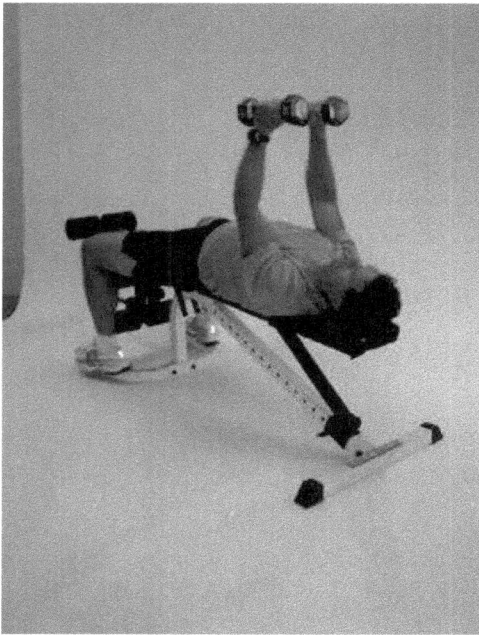

Start

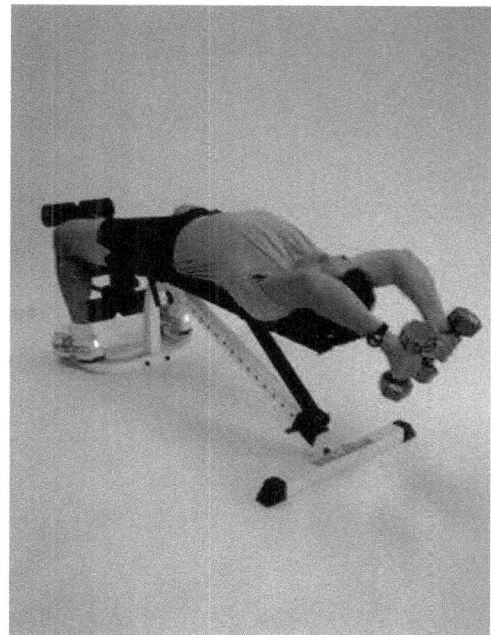

Finish

- Lay flat on a bench, putting your feet up is optional.
- Grip the dumbbells as shown in the picture, weights are pointed up and down. This exercise can also be done holding one dumbbell instead of two.
- Pull the weights up until they are approximately over your chin – your elbows should be slightly bent.
- Lower back to the starting position – get a full stretch according to your own level of flexibility.

Mike's Special Pointer:

Keep your arms bent slightly and keep the angle the same both up and down. Bending the elbows too much brings the triceps into it creating a different exercise.

Calf Raise Machine - Standing

TARGET AREA -   Calves - back of lower legs

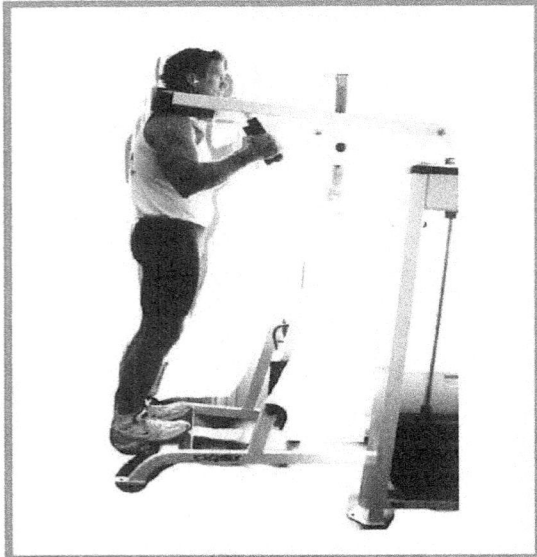

Start

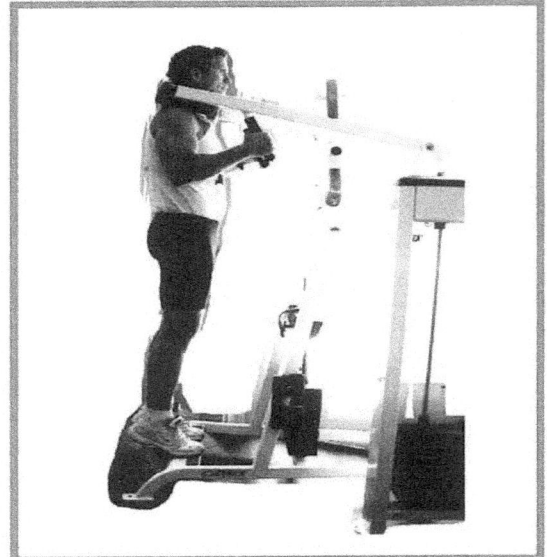

Finish

* Set machine so that you're able to go all the way up and all the way down without the weight stack touching the top or bottom.
* Get under shoulder pads, keep your back straight and lift the weight stack initially by pressing with your legs, not by bending your back.
* Position your feet so that the balls of your feet are on the step, heels hanging over, grab hand grips.
* Allow your calves to stretch fully by bringing your heels as close to the ground as possible, push up onto the balls of your feet as high as possible and pause briefly. Come back to a full stretch.

Mike's Special Pointer:
Keep a very slight bend in your knees while doing this exercise and keep it there for the entire time both up and down. Also, pause at top for at least ½ second for maximum effectiveness.

Bicep Curls: Bar, Close Grip

Target Area – Biceps (front of upper arms)

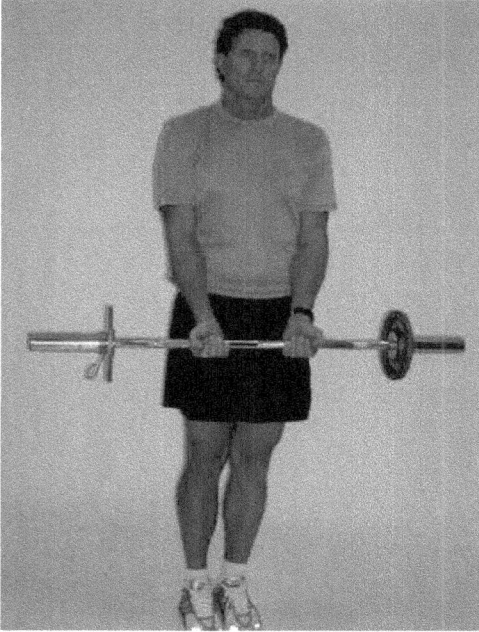

Start

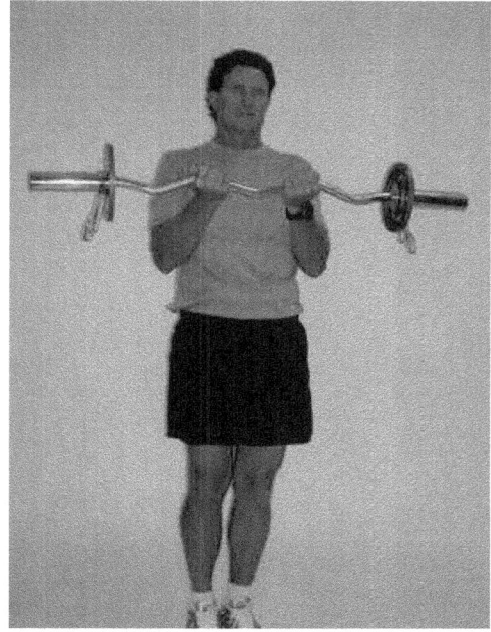

Finish

- Hold a curl bar a little less narrow than shoulder's width, feet apart, soft knees (this means very slightly bent)
- Keeping elbows down, curl arm up to the top of your chest.
- Lower back down to starting position.

Mike's Special Pointer:

Try not to use your back to cheat, as you so commonly see. People do this by leaning back as they curl up. Not only isn't this as effective, but it can be dangerous for your lower back.

Rows - Low Cable - Narrow Grip

TARGET AREA - Latisimus - upper and outer back

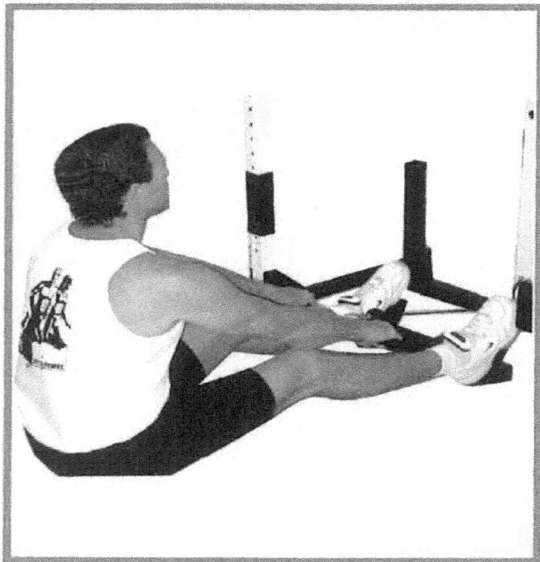

Start

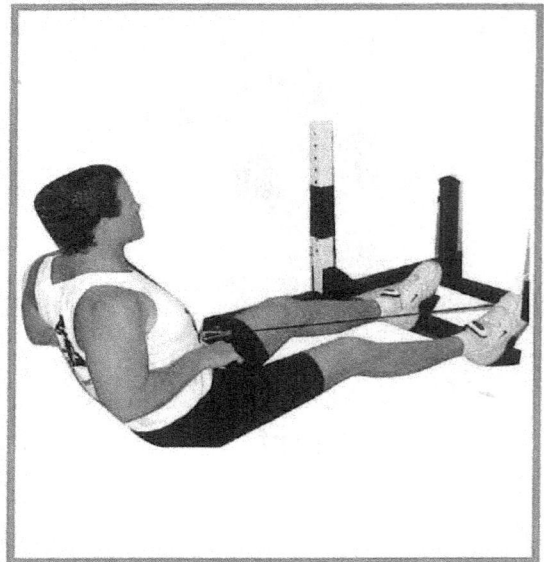

Finish

* Grab the bar narrower than shoulders width with your palms facing down.
* Your back should be flat, and leaning slightly forward in the start position.
* Pull straight back, as you move your back slightly back.
* Pull the bar just above the navel.
* Move your back the other way as you return to the starting position - allow your arms to stretch out.

Mike's Special Pointer:
Don't lean too far back when doing this exercise. You'll notice in the picture very little movement. Also, don't round your back- keep it flat.

Lunges: Stationary

Target Area – Quadriceps and Glutei (front of upper legs and buttocks)

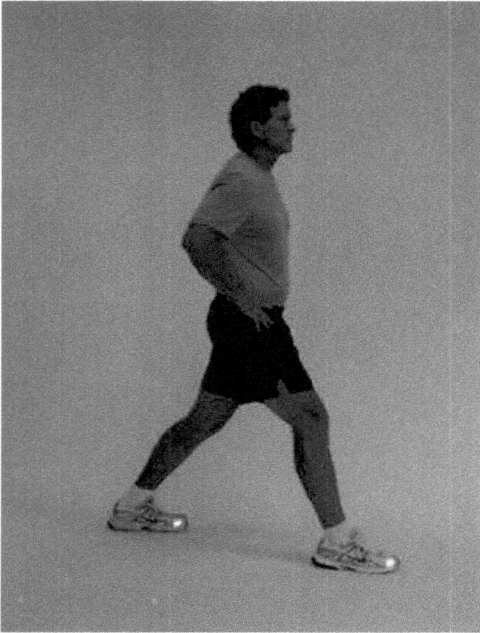

Start

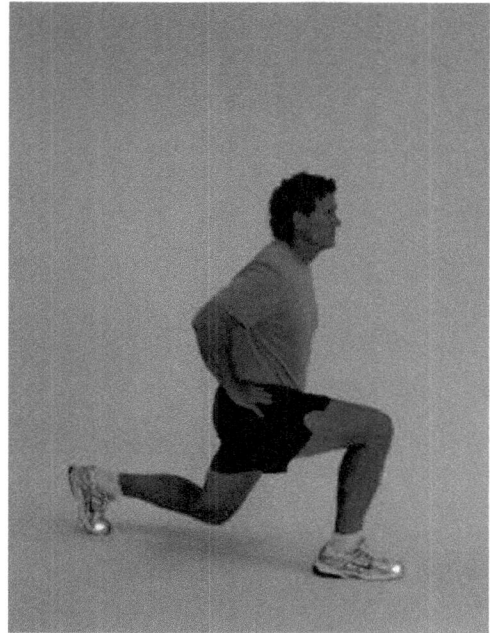

Finish

- To get into the starting position, place one foot well in front of the other with your hands on your hips (or holding weights, if desired).
- Lower yourself down until the back knee almost touches the ground.
- Keeping your front foot in the same place, push back up to the start position. Your feet do not change positions until you are done with the set on that side.
- When you've done all the desired number of repetitions on one leg, switch legs and do the other leg.

Mike's Special Pointer:

Try not to lean forward when doing this exercise. Keep your back straight up and down.

Dumbbell Dead Lifts

Target Area – Glutei, (buttocks and lower back)

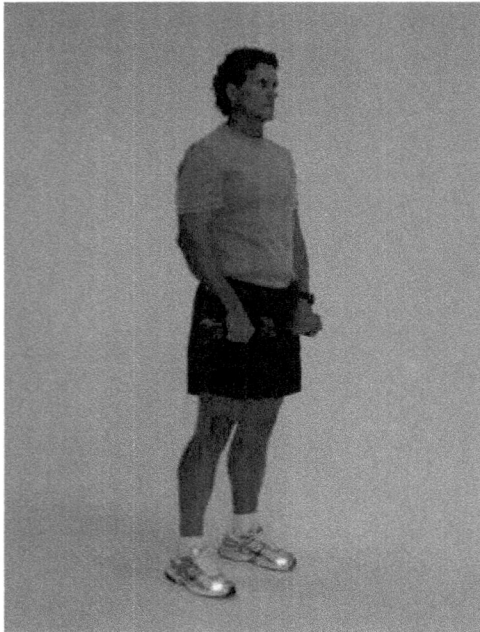

Start

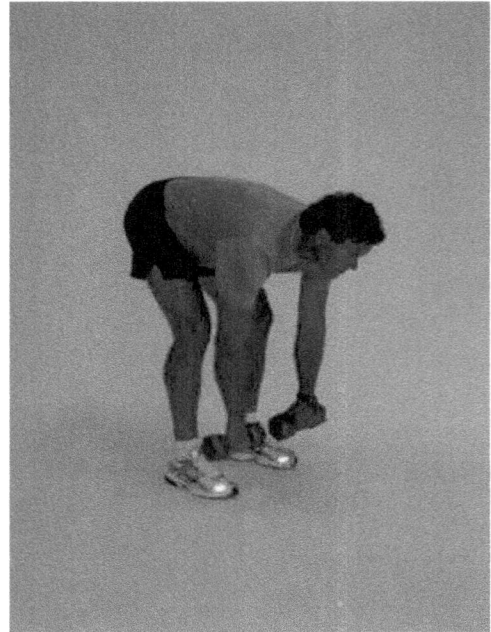

Finish

- Start with feet about shoulder's width, dumbbells at your sides. Bend at the waist and come down until your back is about parallel to the ground.
- As you come down, be sure to keep your back flat, keep your chin up. At the down position, your arms should be hanging straight down. Pull back up to the starting position.
- Come up all the way, but don't lean back at the top.

Mike's Special Pointer:

Be sure to keep your back flat during this exercise, as opposed to rounded. Use a mirror to check your form by standing sideways to the mirror.

Leg Curls - Laying on Stomach

TARGET AREA -   Hamstrings - back of upper legs

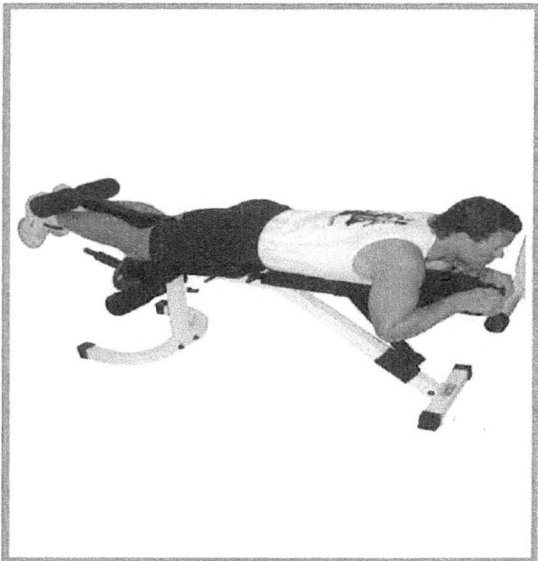

Start

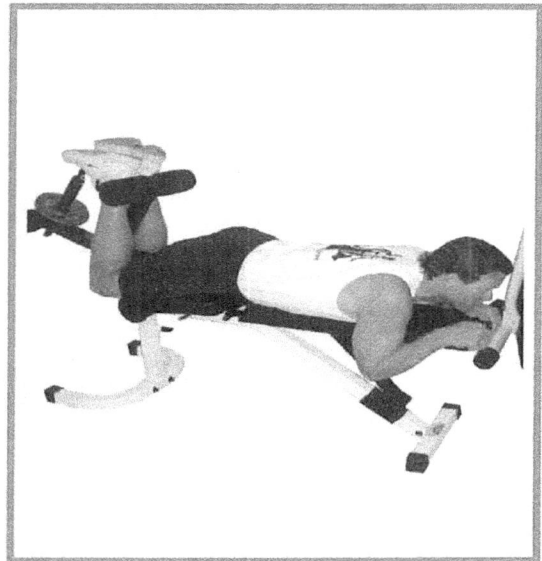

Finish

* Lay face down on leg curl machine, hook your ankles behind the rollers, grab handles loosely.
* Pull your heels towards you buttocks keeping your feet relaxed.
* Come Up as far as you can, try to get to at least a 90 degree bend at the knees.
* Lower the weight back to the starting position.

Mike's Special Pointer:
Be sure to not poke your buttocks up into the air, when doing this exercise. Keep it down! Many people injure their back when they arch their back up off the pad.

Inner Thigh Machine

TARGET AREA -   Inner Thighs

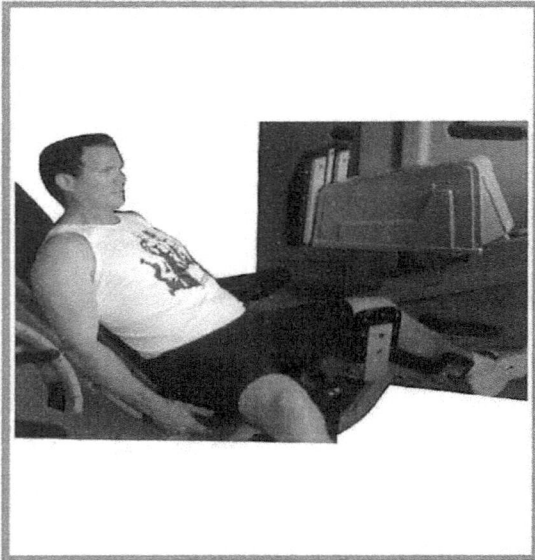

Start

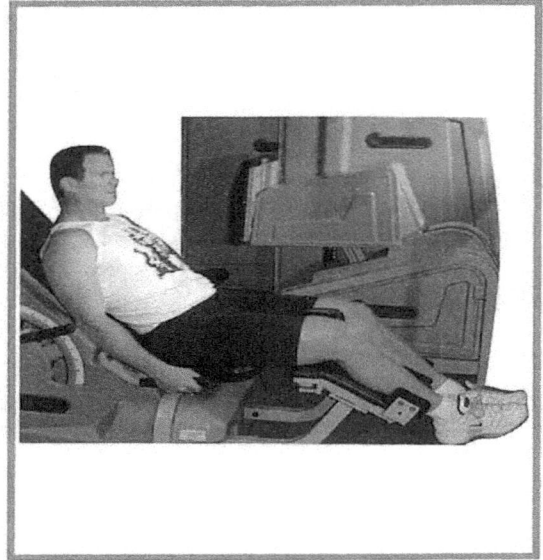

Finish

* Set machine so that you can get a full stretch without the weight touching down in the start position. Sit back in seat, position pads inside the legs.
* Hold onto handles.
* Allow machine to stretch your inner thighs as knees spread further apart.
* Squeeze your legs back together until pads meet in front of you.
* Ease your legs back apart to full stretch.

Mike's Special Pointer:
When doing this exercise, think of pushing with your knees, not your feet. Also, it's important to keep your legs straight up. Don't turn your heels in when pulling together.

Outer Thigh Machine

TARGET AREA -   Outer Thighs

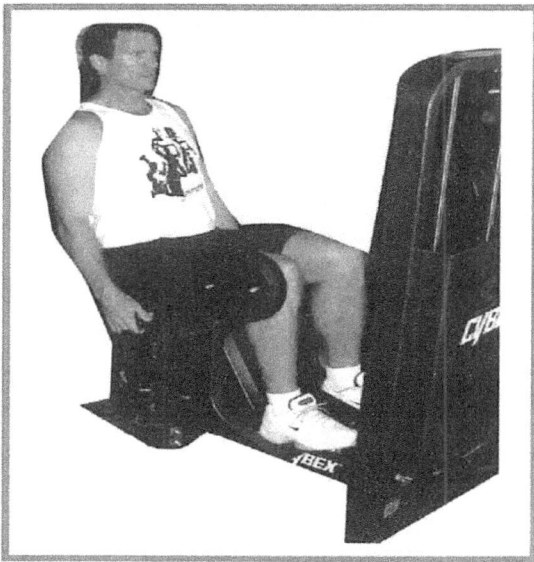

Start

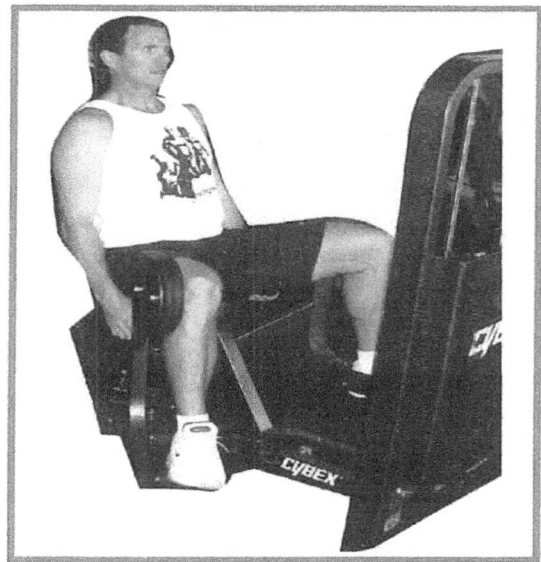

Finish

* Sit in seat, knee pads should be on the outside of your legs.
* Hold hand grips.
* Push out as far as you can, pause, and come back out to start position.

Mike's Special Pointer:
You'll get a lot more out of this exercise if you hold the weight out
in the finish position for at least 1 second. Go out as far as you can,
hold it there, then return slowly.

Concentration Curls

Biceps - front of upper arms

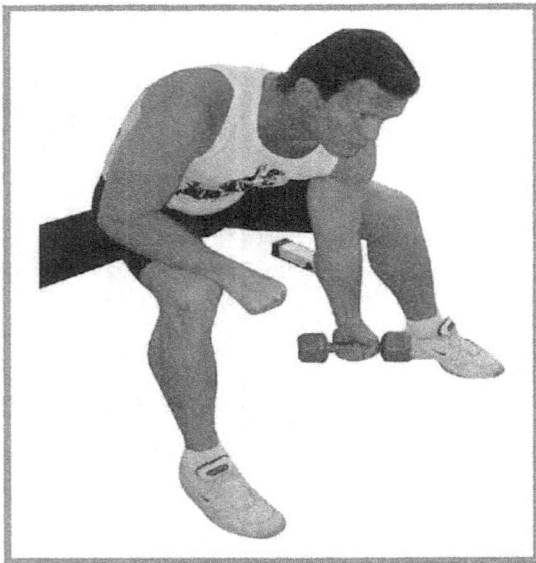

Start

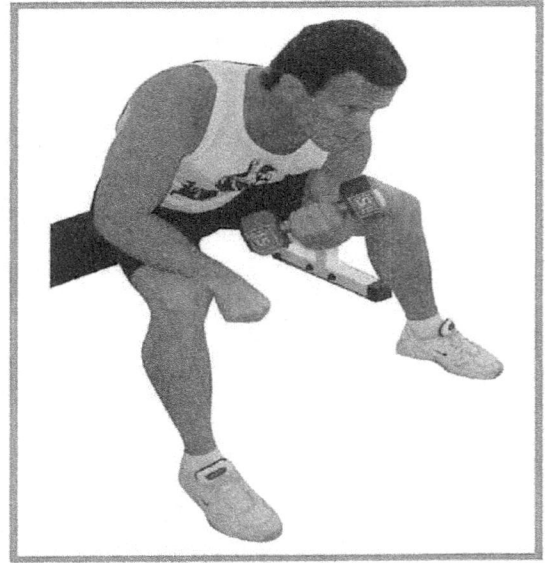

Finish

* Sit sideways on a bench or chair and spread your legs.
* Put non-working arm so that it supports upper body weight just above the knee.
* Hang the working arm down, palm facing towards your other leg, back of upper arm braced against the inside of your leg near your knee.
* Curl the weight up, keeping your upper body steady- go as high as you can.
* Lower the weight back down to start position.

Mike's Special Pointer:
Come all the way down until your arm is straight. Doing bicep curls with a short range of motion can shorten your tendons and make you more prone to injury.

Lower Back Machine

TARGET AREA -   Lower Back

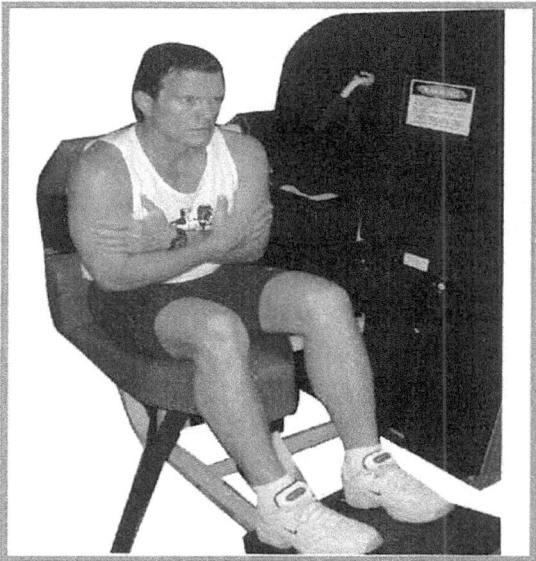

Start

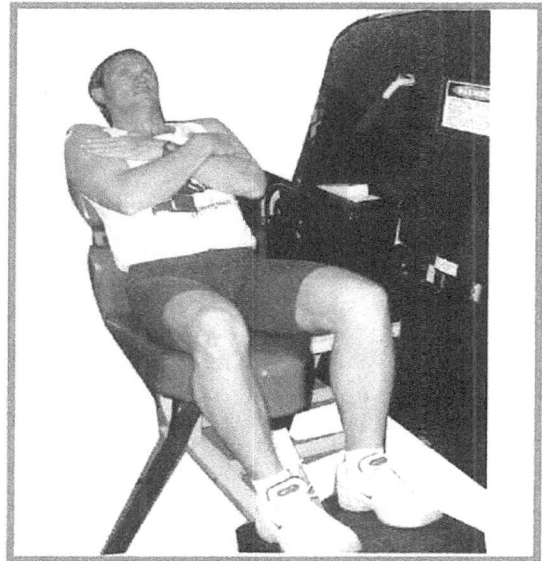

Finish

* Set foot pad so knees are comfortably bent. Sit in machine, cross hands over chest.
* Push back until legs and body are straight or until weight touches at top (depending on which style of machine you use).
* Come forward to a stretch, or until weight touches back down.

Mike's Special Pointer:
Careful on this machine- it 's a good exercise, but don't try and lift heavy at first. Start light, and gradually progress as the weeks pass.

Pain Free Functional Strength Workout - Advanced Female: Chest, Shoulders, Triceps, Abs, Traps

Quick Sheet – Review and Additional Instructions

Before Starting:

* Be sure you have a way to make small increases when using weights or dumbbells less than 50 pounds.

* Take one workout to get your starting weight established for each exercise. For all exercises, find the weight that you can get one set of 10 reps moderately easy.

* Write down all these starting weights on your *Pain Free Functional Strength* workout chart, just above the word "weight".

* Each exercise is explained in detail in the pages that follow your workout chart.

Pain Free Functional Strength: The Workout

* Your first workout – Do 3 sets of 8 reps for each exercise. (Except for the calf raises, abdominal exercises, shoulder shrugs and wrist curls. Instead of doing 8, 9, 10, 11 and 12 reps you will use 11, 12, 13, 14, and 15 reps for these exercises instead)

* Workout Number 2 – do 3 sets of 9 reps

* Workout Number 3 – do 3 sets of 10 reps

* Workout Number 4 – do 3 sets of 11 reps

* Workout Number 5 – do 3 sets of 12 reps

* Workout Number 6 – Increase the weight by only 5 to 10 percent for each exercise. But now drop your reps back to 3 sets of 8

* Workout Number 7 – do 3 sets of 9 reps

* Workout Number 8 – do 3 sets of 10 reps

* Workout Number 9 – do 3 sets of 11 reps

* Workout Number 10 – do 3 sets of 12 reps

* Workout Number 11 - Increase the weights by 5 to 10 percent once again on those exercises that you got 3 sets of 12 on during the last workout. Continue the normal progression on all the other exercises, or use the next 5 workouts to "even it out" (as described in chapter 6)

* Continue as long as you can using this pattern

* *Pain Free Functional Strength* ends on an exercise when you can no longer get the number of reps that the workout calls for 2 workouts in a row.

* For the remaining workouts, continue doing those exercises that came to an end for at least your 3 sets of 8 reps, while working the progression for the remaining exercises. When all the exercises

have come to their anticipated end, you have finished *Pain Free Functional Strength* – Congratulations!

What now? Pick all new exercises and start back at the beginning. Or continue on this workout but decrease the weight by 33% and do 5, 6, and 7 reps instead of 8 through 12.

Additional Exercises: (not to be done using the *Pain Free Functional Strength* system)

Crunches, Crunches - Cross Elbow Knee Raise, Toe Touches (alternating), Bicycle Sit-ups
Do 1 or 2 sets of each, 10 – 25 reps for each exercise. Start moderately and build up the reps and sets gradually.

Workout Chart - For 8, 9, 10, 11 and 12 reps – Advanced Female: Chest, Shoulders, Triceps, Abs, Traps

(Cross off rep counts as you progress through workouts)

Exercise #1: Dumbbell Bench Press	Weight: _____ 8,9,10,11,12 _____ 8,9,10,11,12 _____ 8,9,10,11,12	_____ 8,9,10,11,12 _____ 8,9,10,11,12 _____ 8,9,10,11,12	_____ 8,9,10,11,12 _____ 8,9,10,11,12 _____ 8,9,10,11,12
Exercise #2: Dumbbell Lateral raise, Bent Over Seated (Do 2 sets)	Weight: _____ 8,9,10,11,12 _____ 8,9,10,11,12 _____ 8,9,10,11,12	_____ 8,9,10,11,12 _____ 8,9,10,11,12 _____ 8,9,10,11,12	_____ 8,9,10,11,12 _____ 8,9,10,11,12 _____ 8,9,10,11,12
Exercise #3: Dumbbell Triceps Ext. On Back	Weight: _____ 8,9,10,11,12 _____ 8,9,10,11,12 _____ 8,9,10,11,12	_____ 8,9,10,11,12 _____ 8,9,10,11,12 _____ 8,9,10,11,12	_____ 8,9,10,11,12 _____ 8,9,10,11,12 _____ 8,9,10,11,12
Exercise #4: Abdominal Machine (Do 10,11,12,13,14 reps)	Weight: _____ 10,11,12,13,14 _____ 10,11,12,13,14 _____ 10,11,12,13,14	_____ 10,11,12,13,14 _____ 10,11,12,13,14 _____ 10,11,12,13,14	_____ 10,11,12,13,14 _____ 10,11,12,13,14 _____ 10,11,12,13,14
Exercise #5: Dumbbell Military Press Standing, Twist	Weight: _____ 8,9,10,11,12 _____ 8,9,10,11,12 _____ 8,9,10,11,12	_____ 8,9,10,11,12 _____ 8,9,10,11,12 _____ 8,9,10,11,12	_____ 8,9,10,11,12 _____ 8,9,10,11,12 _____ 8,9,10,11,12
Exercise #6: Dumbbell Shrugs (Do 10,11,12,13,14 reps)	Weight: _____ 10,11,12,13,14 _____ 10,11,12,13,14 _____ 10,11,12,13,14	_____ 10,11,12,13,14 _____ 10,11,12,13,14 _____ 10,11,12,13,14	_____ 10,11,12,13,14 _____ 10,11,12,13,14 _____ 10,11,12,13,14
Exercise #7: Chest Flies, Cable	Weight: _____ 8,9,10,11,12 _____ 8,9,10,11,12 _____ 8,9,10,11,12	_____ 8,9,10,11,12 _____ 8,9,10,11,12 _____ 8,9,10,11,12	_____ 8,9,10,11,12 _____ 8,9,10,11,12 _____ 8,9,10,11,12
Exercise #8: Dumbbell Kickbacks	Weight: _____ 8,9,10,11,12 _____ 8,9,10,11,12 _____ 8,9,10,11,12	_____ 8,9,10,11,12 _____ 8,9,10,11,12 _____ 8,9,10,11,12	_____ 8,9,10,11,12 _____ 8,9,10,11,12 _____ 8,9,10,11,12
Exercise #9: Dips, Assisted	Weight: _____ 8,9,10,11,12 _____ 8,9,10,11,12 _____ 8,9,10,11,12	_____ 8,9,10,11,12 _____ 8,9,10,11,12 _____ 8,9,10,11,12	_____ 8,9,10,11,12 _____ 8,9,10,11,12 _____ 8,9,10,11,12

Additional Exercises:

Crunches, Crunches - Cross Elbow Knee Raise, Toe Touches (alternating), Bicycle Sit-ups

Do 1 or 2 sets of each, 10 – 25 reps for each exercise. Start moderately and build up the reps and sets gradually.

Dumbbell Bench Press

Target Area – Pectorals (chest)

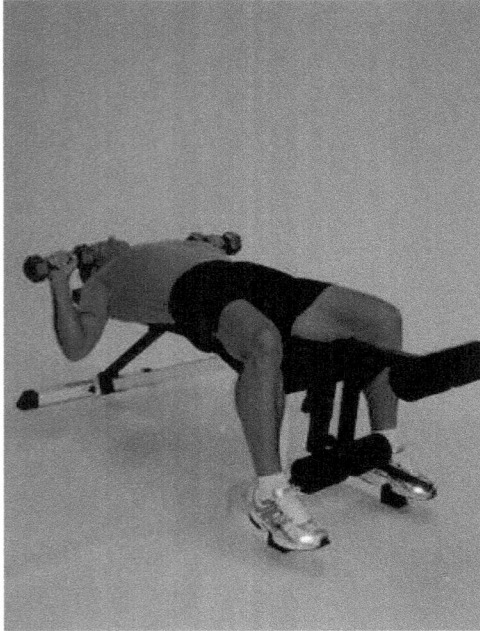

Start

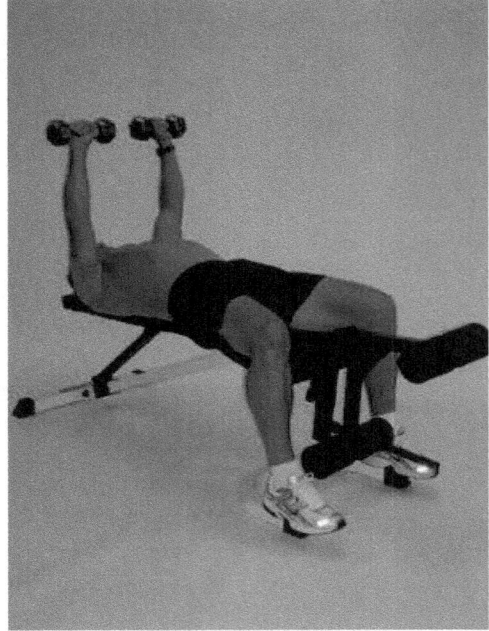

Finish

- Lay flat on your back, putting your feet up is optional.
- Start with the weights wider than your shoulders, elbows at or slightly below the bench.
- Push up and allow the weights to come close together at the top without touching.
- Don't lock out your elbows.
- Come back down to the start position, but don't let your forearms angle out – keep them straight up.

Mike's Special Pointer:

When pushing up, it's OK if your elbows are slightly forward. Many people can develop shoulder injuries if they try and force their elbows way back while doing the exercise.

Dumbbell Lateral Raise - Bent Over - Seated

TARGET AREA -   Deltoids - back of shoulders

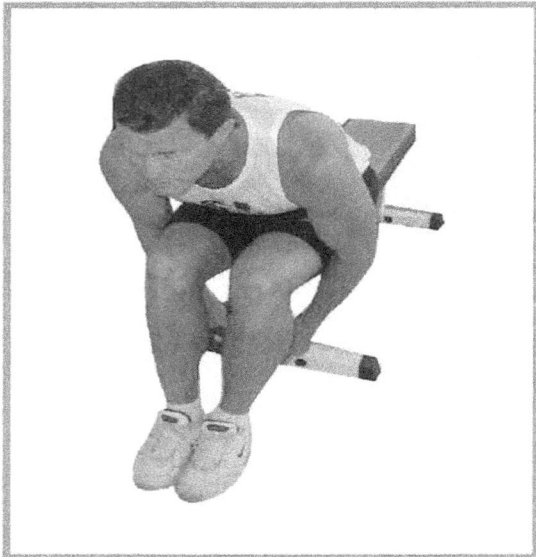

Start

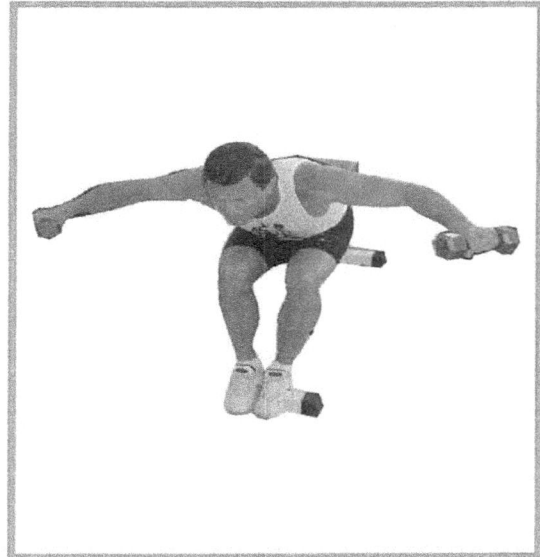

Finish

* Sit on the edge of a bench or on a chair, bend over and hold weights under legs, chin up, back flat.
* Extend your arms out and come up to where forearms are pointed to the sides, but slightly forward.
* Lower back down to start position under legs.

Mike's Special Pointer:
Stay down while doing this exercise. The tendency is to sit more upright, changing the target area of the exercise.

Dumbbell Triceps Extension: On Back

Target Area – Triceps (back of upper arms)

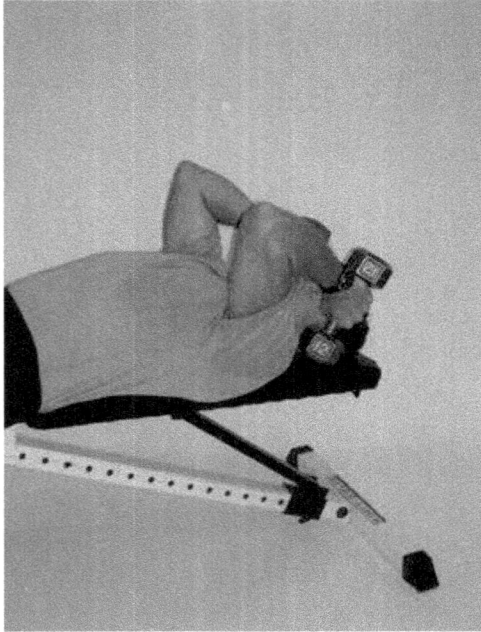

Start

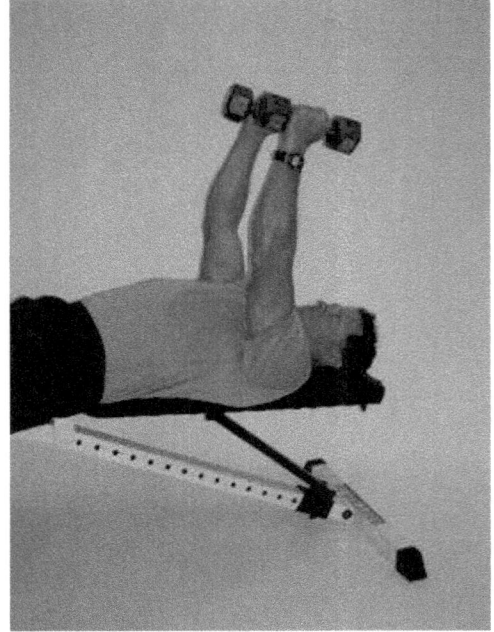

Finish

- Lay flat on a bench, knees up or down according to your preference, dumbbells held straight up, palms facing towards each other.
- Keeping elbows in and up, lower the weights so your hands come approximately to your ears.
- Push back up to the start position.

Mike's Special Pointer:

Keep those elbows in the same place. They tend to want to move backwards and forwards as you do the movements. Don't let that happen though – keep them stationary.

Abdominal Machine

TARGET AREA -   Abdominals - front of torso

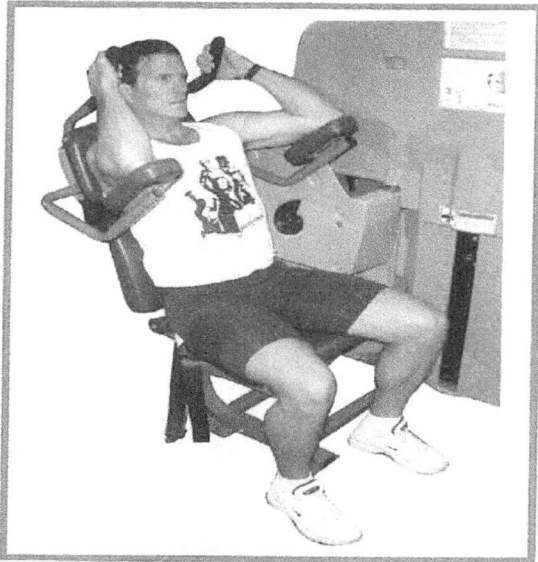
Start

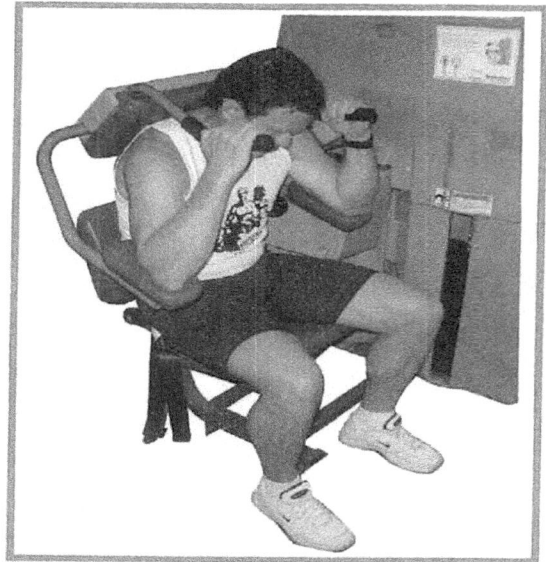
Finish

* Set seat so that your navel is about in line with axis of rotating arm of machine.
* Sit in seat, grab handles (if available), feet flat on floor, sit upright.
* Using your abdominal muscles, pull forward and then down.
* Return to starting position.

Mike's Special Pointer:
Don't allow your back to come out of the seat- keep it back at all times.

Dumbbell Military Press (Standing) - Twisting

TARGET AREA -   Deltoids - shoulders

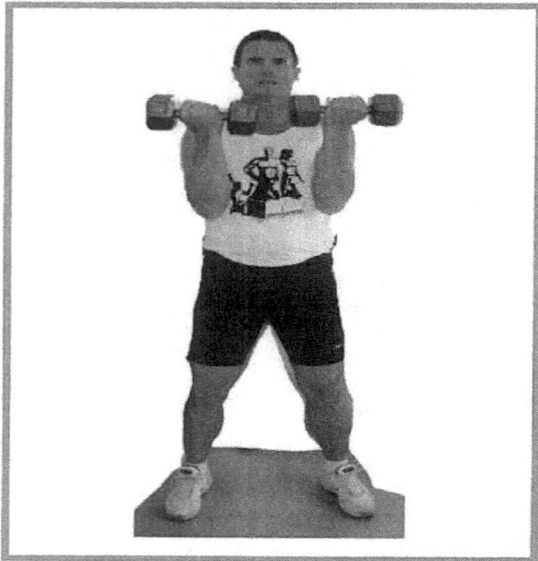

Start

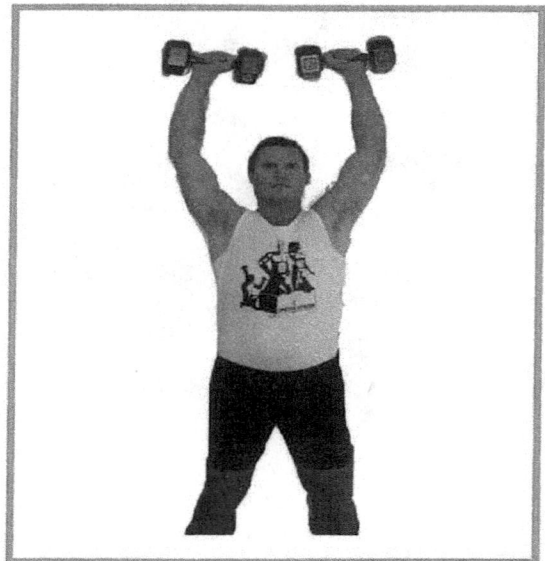

Finish

* This exercise can be done either sitting or standing (as illustrated above).
* Hold the weights so palms face you, hands just below chin level.
* Push up and as you do rotate the dumbbells so that the palms turn towards each other and then finally end up palms facing forward once you have arrived at the top.
* Your knees should be slightly bent but not locked
* Come back to the start position, rotate the opposite way as on the way up.

Mike's Special Pointer:
Be careful not to hit yourself with the dumbbells as you rotate your arms. Check in the mirror to make sure you are well in the clear.

175

Dumbbell Shrugs

Target Area: Trapezius (upper back)

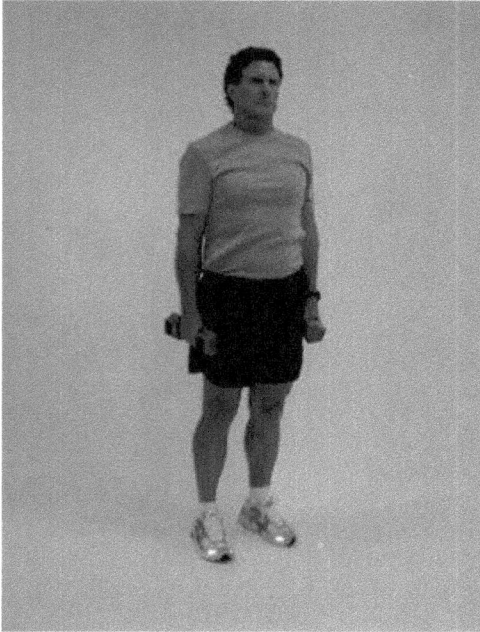

Start

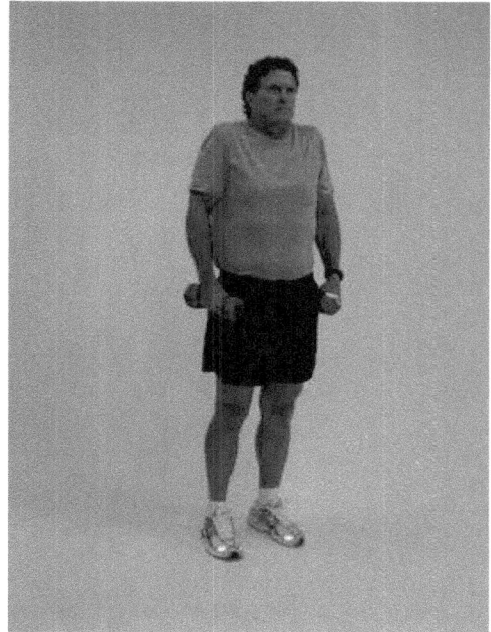

Finish

- Stand holding dumbbells at your sides, feet close together, knees slightly bent, palms facing in.
- Shrug your shoulders up as high as you can with hardly any bend of the elbows.
- Come back down to a full stretch at the bottom.

Mike's Special Pointer:

Dumbbell shrugs have one advantage over regular bar shrugs. You can move the weight forward or backwards a little until you feel it the best, whereas the bar only allows you one angle.

Chest Flies: Cable

Target Area – Pectorals (chest)

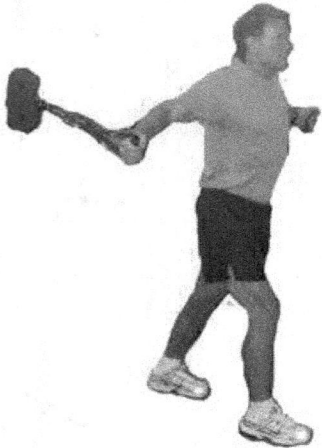

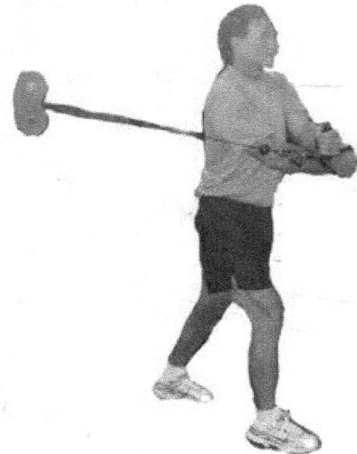

Start   **Finish**

- Put handles on upper part of cable machine.
- Grab one handle, move over sideways far enough to grab other handle, come back to center, feet nearly together, knees bent slightly, arms extended up and out.
- With palms forward in start position, pull handles in front of you until they cross, keep elbows bent slightly the whole time.
- Come back up to a stretch.

Mike's Special Pointer:

I like to cross my hands differently after each repetition, right over left, left over right, etc. This ensures equal use of the muscles.

Dumbbell Kickbacks

Target Area – Triceps (back of upper arms)

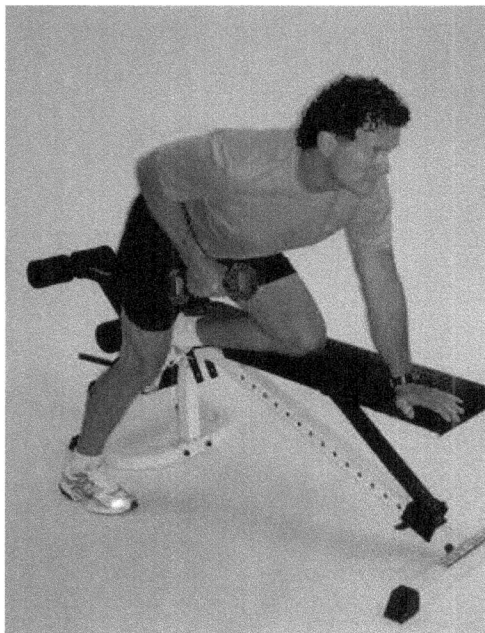

Start

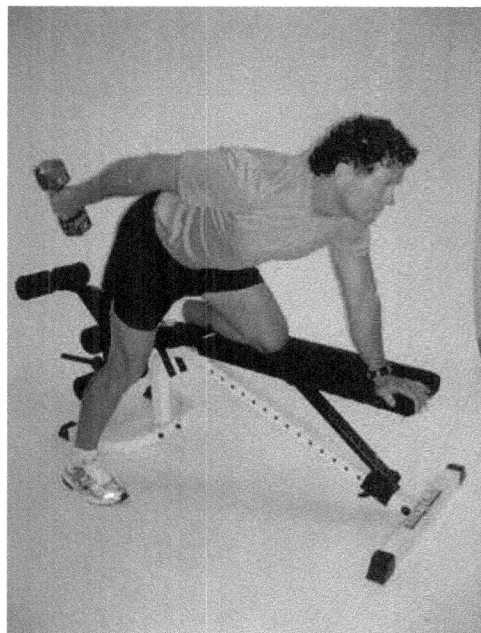

Finish

- Place your non-working hand and your knee (same side as non-working hand) firmly on a bench.
- Your other leg should be extended back for support.
- Start with the dumbbell under your shoulder, elbow back.
- Keeping your elbow high, extend your hand back and turn it slightly so your palm almost faces the ceiling at full extension.
- Come back to start position, do all your reps and repeat on the other side.

Mike's Special Pointer:

Many people do kickbacks without the little twist on the way up. But give this a try and you'll see this trick works your triceps a lot harder.

Dips - Assisted

<u>TARGET AREA -</u>　　　Pectorals & Triceps - chest and back of upper arms

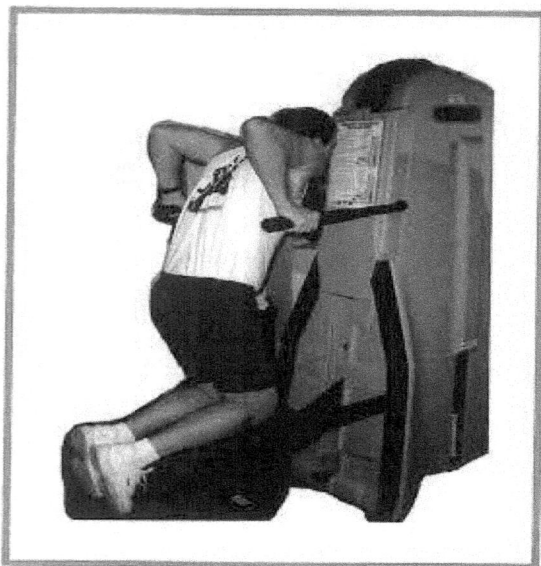

Start

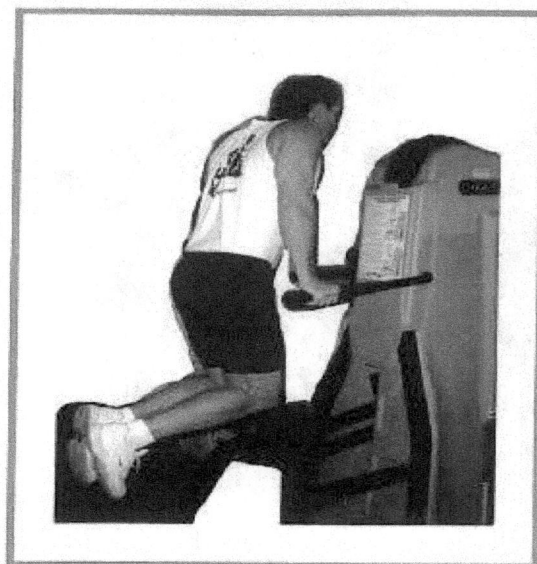

Finish

* Set weight with the weight stack pin, the more weight you use the easier the exercise.
* Grab bars at your sides with palms facing in, step or kneel onto the assisting pad, extend your arms fully without locking your elbows.
* Keeping elbows back, come down into a stretch.
* Push back up to start position.

Mike's Special Pointer:
To work your triceps harder, keep your elbows back when coming down and pushing up. It's OK to lean slightly forward.

Crunches

Target Area – Abdominals (front of torso)

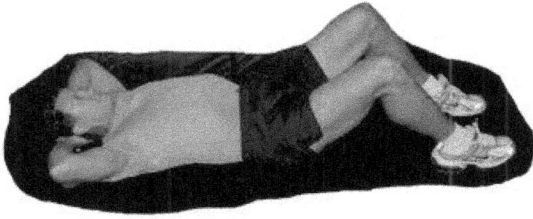
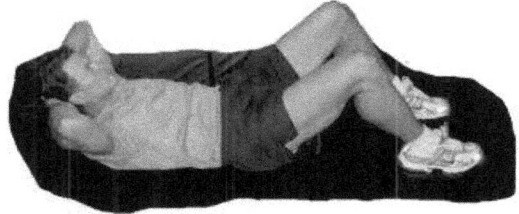

Start   **Finish**

- Lay flat on a mat or the floor, keep your lower back pressed down against the floor, raise knees but keep your feet flat on the floor.
- Interlace your fingers behind your head, point your elbows mostly out to the sides.
- Using your abdominal muscles, curl up as you press your lower back further down into the floor.
- Pause at the top for a moment at the top, and then return back to the start position.

Mike's Special Pointer:

How high you come up when doing crunches makes a big difference on the effectiveness of the exercise. Try to actually get your shoulder blades up off the floor when in the finish position.

Crunches: Cross Elbow-Knee

Target Area – Abdominals and Oblique's (front and sides of torso)

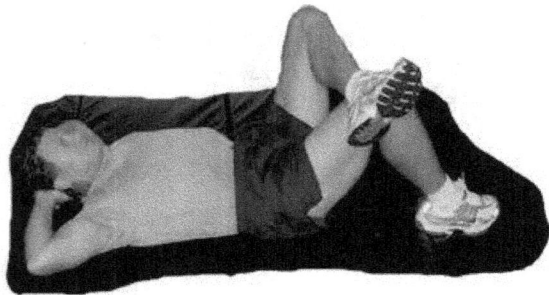 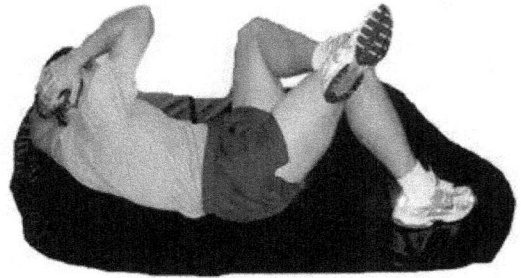

Start   **Finish**

- Lay on the floor, fingers clasped under the base of your head.
- Put one ankle up on your opposite knee.
- Come up with one elbow towards the knee that's up on the opposite side, keep your other elbow down on the floor.
- Come up and over, you don't want to actually touch your elbow to your knee.
- Come back down to the start position, finish your reps, then change to the other side.

Mike's Special Pointer:

Some people do like to make contact with the elbow to the knee, but that changes the exercise. Keeping your opposite elbow down forces you to use more of the sides of your abdominals.

Toe Touches: Alternating

Target Area: Gluteal (buttocks), Oblique (sides)

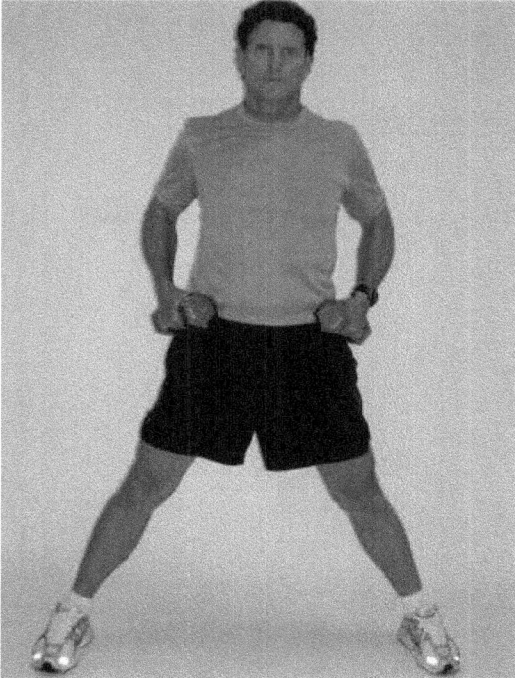

Start

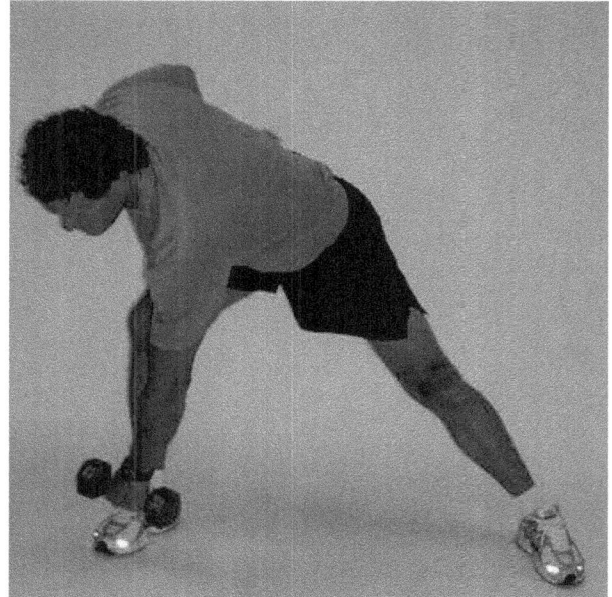

Finish

- Position your feet wider than shoulder's width, toes pointed forward, hands with or without dumbbells.
- Take one hand and go towards your opposite foot while twisting and lowering your upper body.
- The knee that you're bending towards should bend slightly. Bring your hand to, or at least near your toes.
- Come back up to the starting position and repeat side to side in an alternating fashion.

Mike's Special Pointer:

Come all the way back up when you come to the top, so that you're standing straight up in between going from side to side.

Sit Ups - Bicycle

<u>TARGET AREA -</u>   <u>Abdominals & Obliques - front & sides of torso</u>

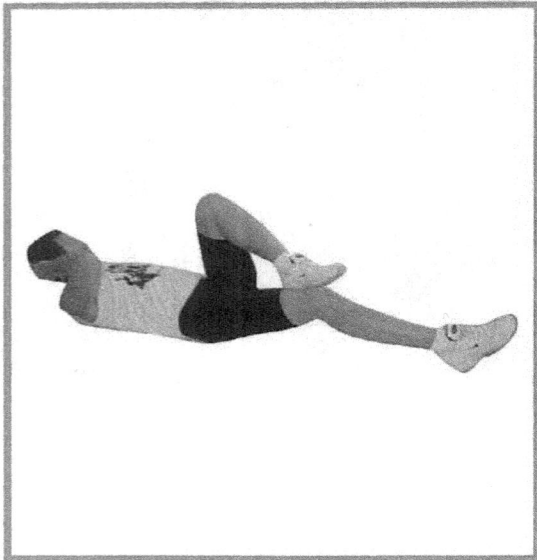

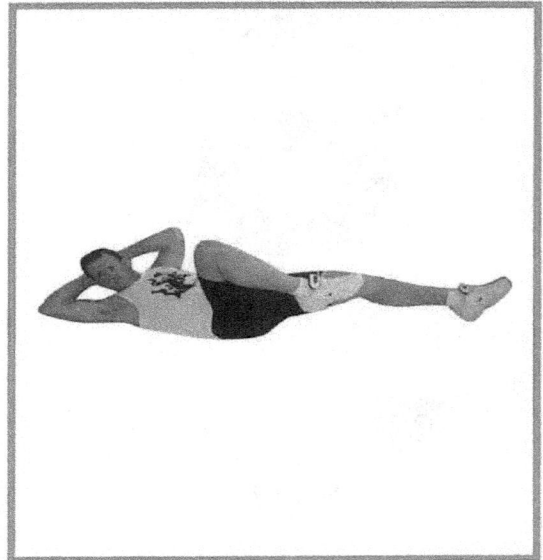

Start   Finish

*   Lay flat on your back on the floor or a mat, lightly clasp your fingers behind your head, raise both feet off the floor with knees slightly bent.
*   Bring one knee up as the opposite elbow turns toward it.
*   Stop well short of the elbow touching the knee.
*   Next, bring the other leg in as the original leg extends out.
*   While this is happening you're pivoting your upper body the other way so that your other elbow is moving towards your opposite knee.
*   Keep crisscrossing until you've done the desired number of repetitions.

Mike's Special Pointer:

Don't swing your shoulders side to side on the floor. Think of a pivot rod attached to the top of your head, not allowing your head to move all around- only pivot. That's the action you're looking for.

The following are blank workout charts for your convenience. Feel free to photocopy them as needed for your workouts

Additional Pain Free Functional Strength Workout Chart Blanks:

Blank Workout Chart for 8, 9, 10, 11 and 12 Reps

Exercise #1	Weight:	8,9,10,11,12	8,9,10,11,12	8,9,10,11,12
		8,9,10,11,12	8,9,10,11,12	8,9,10,11,12
		8,9,10,11,12	8,9,10,11,12	8,9,10,11,12
Exercise #2	Weight:	8,9,10,11,12	8,9,10,11,12	8,9,10,11,12
		8,9,10,11,12	8,9,10,11,12	8,9,10,11,12
		8,9,10,11,12	8,9,10,11,12	8,9,10,11,12
Exercise #3	Weight:	8,9,10,11,12	8,9,10,11,12	8,9,10,11,12
		8,9,10,11,12	8,9,10,11,12	8,9,10,11,12
		8,9,10,11,12	8,9,10,11,12	8,9,10,11,12
Exercise #4	Weight:	8,9,10,11,12	8,9,10,11,12	8,9,10,11,12
		8,9,10,11,12	8,9,10,11,12	8,9,10,11,12
		8,9,10,11,12	8,9,10,11,12	8,9,10,11,12
Exercise #5	Weight:	8,9,10,11,12	8,9,10,11,12	8,9,10,11,12
		8,9,10,11,12	8,9,10,11,12	8,9,10,11,12
		8,9,10,11,12	8,9,10,11,12	8,9,10,11,12
Exercise #6	Weight:	8,9,10,11,12	8,9,10,11,12	8,9,10,11,12
		8,9,10,11,12	8,9,10,11,12	8,9,10,11,12
		8,9,10,11,12	8,9,10,11,12	8,9,10,11,12
Exercise #7	Weight:	8,9,10,11,12	8,9,10,11,12	8,9,10,11,12
		8,9,10,11,12	8,9,10,11,12	8,9,10,11,12
		8,9,10,11,12	8,9,10,11,12	8,9,10,11,12
Exercise #8	Weight:	8,9,10,11,12	8,9,10,11,12	8,9,10,11,12
		8,9,10,11,12	8,9,10,11,12	8,9,10,11,12
		8,9,10,11,12	8,9,10,11,12	8,9,10,11,12
Exercise #9	Weight:	8,9,10,11,12	8,9,10,11,12	8,9,10,11,12
		8,9,10,11,12	8,9,10,11,12	8,9,10,11,12
		8,9,10,11,12	8,9,10,11,12	8,9,10,11,12
Exercise #10	Weight:	8,9,10,11,12	8,9,10,11,12	8,9,10,11,12
		8,9,10,11,12	8,9,10,11,12	8,9,10,11,12
		8,9,10,11,12	8,9,10,11,12	8,9,10,11,12

Copyright Pain Free Functional Strength Mike Spotts Fitness, all rights reserved.

Blank Workout Chart for 5, 6, and 7 Reps

Exercise #1	**Weight:** _____ 5,6,7 _____ 5,6,7 _____ 5,6,7	_____ 5,6,7 _____ 5,6,7 _____ 5,6,7	_____ 5,6,7 _____ 5,6,7 _____ 5,6,7
Exercise #2	**Weight:** _____ 5,6,7 _____ 5,6,7 _____ 5,6,7	_____ 5,6,7 _____ 5,6,7 _____ 5,6,7	_____ 5,6,7 _____ 5,6,7 _____ 5,6,7
Exercise #3	**Weight:** _____ 5,6,7 _____ 5,6,7 _____ 5,6,7	_____ 5,6,7 _____ 5,6,7 _____ 5,6,7	_____ 5,6,7 _____ 5,6,7 _____ 5,6,7
Exercise #4	**Weight:** _____ 5,6,7 _____ 5,6,7 _____ 5,6,7	_____ 5,6,7 _____ 5,6,7 _____ 5,6,7	_____ 5,6,7 _____ 5,6,7 _____ 5,6,7
Exercise #5	**Weight:** _____ 5,6,7 _____ 5,6,7 _____ 5,6,7	_____ 5,6,7 _____ 5,6,7 _____ 5,6,7	_____ 5,6,7 _____ 5,6,7 _____ 5,6,7
Exercise #6	**Weight:** _____ 5,6,7 _____ 5,6,7 _____ 5,6,7	_____ 5,6,7 _____ 5,6,7 _____ 5,6,7	_____ 5,6,7 _____ 5,6,7 _____ 5,6,7
Exercise #7	**Weight:** _____ 5,6,7 _____ 5,6,7 _____ 5,6,7	_____ 5,6,7 _____ 5,6,7 _____ 5,6,7	_____ 5,6,7 _____ 5,6,7 _____ 5,6,7
Exercise #8	**Weight:** _____ 5,6,7 _____ 5,6,7 _____ 5,6,7	_____ 5,6,7 _____ 5,6,7 _____ 5,6,7	_____ 5,6,7 _____ 5,6,7 _____ 5,6,7
Exercise #9	**Weight:** _____ 5,6,7 _____ 5,6,7 _____ 5,6,7	_____ 5,6,7 _____ 5,6,7 _____ 5,6,7	_____ 5,6,7 _____ 5,6,7 _____ 5,6,7
Exercise #10	**Weight:** 5,6,7 5,6,7 5,6,7	5,6,7 5,6,7 5,6,7	5,6,7 5,6,7 5,6,7

Copyright Pain Free Functional Strength, Mike Spotts Fitness, all rights reserved.

Blank Workout Chart for 2, 3, and 4 Reps

Exercise #1	**Weight:** _____ 2,3,4 _____ 2,3,4 _____ 2,3,4	_____ 2,3,4 _____ 2,3,4 _____ 2,3,4	_____ 2,3,4 _____ 2,3,4 _____ 2,3,4
Exercise #2	**Weight:** _____ 2,3,4 _____ 2,3,4 _____ 2,3,4	_____ 2,3,4 _____ 2,3,4 _____ 2,3,4	_____ 2,3,4 _____ 2,3,4 _____ 2,3,4
Exercise #3	**Weight:** _____ 2,3,4 _____ 2,3,4 _____ 2,3,4	_____ 2,3,4 _____ 2,3,4 _____ 2,3,4	_____ 2,3,4 _____ 2,3,4 _____ 2,3,4
Exercise #4	**Weight:** _____ 2,3,4 _____ 2,3,4 _____ 2,3,4	_____ 2,3,4 _____ 2,3,4 _____ 2,3,4	_____ 2,3,4 _____ 2,3,4 _____ 2,3,4
Exercise #5	**Weight:** _____ 2,3,4 _____ 2,3,4 _____ 2,3,4	_____ 2,3,4 _____ 2,3,4 _____ 2,3,4	_____ 2,3,4 _____ 2,3,4 _____ 2,3,4
Exercise #6	**Weight:** _____ 2,3,4 _____ 2,3,4 _____ 2,3,4	_____ 2,3,4 _____ 2,3,4 _____ 2,3,4	_____ 2,3,4 _____ 2,3,4 _____ 2,3,4
Exercise #7	**Weight:** _____ 2,3,4 _____ 2,3,4 _____ 2,3,4	_____ 2,3,4 _____ 2,3,4 _____ 2,3,4	_____ 2,3,4 _____ 2,3,4 _____ 2,3,4
Exercise #8	**Weight:** _____ 2,3,4 _____ 2,3,4 _____ 2,3,4	_____ 2,3,4 _____ 2,3,4 _____ 2,3,4	_____ 2,3,4 _____ 2,3,4 _____ 2,3,4
Exercise #9	**Weight:** _____ 2,3,4 _____ 2,3,4 _____ 2,3,4	_____ 2,3,4 _____ 2,3,4 _____ 2,3,4	_____ 2,3,4 _____ 2,3,4 _____ 2,3,4
Exercise #10	**Weight:** _____ 2,3,4 _____ 2,3,4 _____ 2,3,4	_____ 2,3,4 _____ 2,3,4 _____ 2,3,4	_____ 2,3,4 _____ 2,3,4 _____ 2,3,4

Copyright Pain Free Functional Strength, Mike Spotts Fitness, all rights reserved.

www.ingramcontent.com/pod-product-compliance
Lightning Source LLC
Chambersburg PA
CBHW081359270326
41930CB00015B/3360